# PERSPECTIVES ON CANCER

## STORIES OF HEALING, HOPE & RESILIENCE

## TIM SOHN

# ABOUT THE AUTHOR
## TIM SOHN

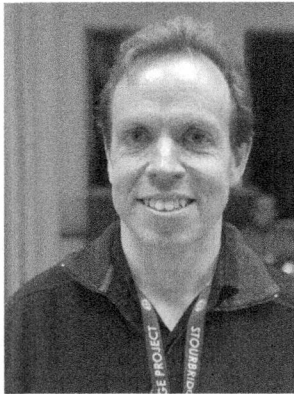

Tim Sohn is a resilient 17-year chronic myeloid leukemia warrior whose cancer came back in 2023. He has an unwavering commitment to support cancer patients, survivors and supporters worldwide. As the host of the groundbreaking weekly livestreamed show, Showing Up: Perspectives On Cancer, Tim created a safe space where cancer survivors and cancer supporters come together to share their stories and connect, as well as find resources that provide healing, hope, and resilience.

Tim's contributions to cancer advocacy have been recognized by the Leukemia & Lymphoma Society, and he was honored with the Mission Award in 2022. As part of his Man & Woman of the Year campaign, Tim organized a 24-hour livestream fundraiser along with his volunteer team and 14 livestreamers from around the world.

With unwavering determination, Tim also hosts annual Showing Up: Perspectives On Cancer In-Person events. This groundbreaking in-person gathering is a testament to his commitment to making a difference in the lives of those affected by cancer.

Through advocacy work, Tim aims to dispel the feelings of isolation and despair that often accompany a cancer diagnosis, and to offer a beacon of hope to those who may be struggling.

He is a true inspiration to cancer patients, survivors and supporters worldwide, as he encourages them to share their stories when they feel ready and reminds them that they are not alone in their journeys.

For more information: PerspectivesOnCancer.com
LinkedIn: @timsohn
Email: tim@sohnsocialmediasolutions.com

# ACKNOWLEDGMENTS

I want to thank from the bottom of my heart all the contributors to this book who have so courageously shared their and their loved ones' cancer stories:

Shannon Lee-Sin

Amanda Rose Ferraro

Anna Tower-Kövesdi

Joe Tower

Ashok Bhattacharya

Branwyn Lee

Dianne Jackson

Josh Tehan

Kim Dunphy

Pamela Formica

Russ Hedge

Sayen Gates

Terry Tucker

Zoraida Morales

# CONTENTS

## DEDICATION

*I dedicate this book to Steve Sullivan, one of the people who inspired me to share my cancer story. He was a 35+ year survivor of acute leukemia. RIP Steve. Love you!*

# 1

# WELCOME, AND MY STORY ON STEROIDS

## BY TIM SOHN

A s I'm writing this, I'm sitting in the waiting area at Geisinger Wyoming Valley Henry Cancer Center in Wilkes-Barre, Pa. But I'm not here for cancer. I'm here for chronic migraine treatment.

Let me back up a little bit. I arrived at Wilkes-Barre last night. My wife and kiddos dropped me off for the three-day adventure (OK, that might be a little bit over hyped). I am here to receive three days of infusions of steroids, saline (for hydration), magnesium and some anti-migraine medications. About six hours a day for three days. (I'm a restless person, so sitting for a long time is a challenge, but so is dealing with migraines on a daily basis, so this is well worth it...)

I've been struggling with migraines for nine years on and off. Recently, they have gotten to the point that there are times I cannot work or live life to the fullest, which is my priority right now, after surviving chronic leukemia for 17 years.

The night we arrived at the hotel, the girls and I went swimming. Honestly, when my wife first mentioned the concept of having the girls go swimming, I didn't like the idea. I thought of these three days as an opportunity for ME to focus on MY health.

But then I reflected on how important it is to find happiness even in a challenging health journey, whether it be migraines, cancer or another adversity.

I'm so glad the girls and I went swimming. We had so much fun!!!

That night I barely slept – I tossed and turned. I was nervous – I didn't know what to expect. I had never had infusions before.

The following morning, I had breakfast at the hotel before heading over – a Western omelet, turkey sausage and coffee. I was really living it up!

Then I called an Uber – I had an enjoyable conversation with the driver. I like to talk to Uber drivers. I would say overall since COVID, I am much less a people-y person, but when I do have the opportunity, I dive in. Everybody has a story – sometimes we can relate to it, sometimes we can't, sometimes we learn something, sometimes we don't, sometimes we laugh, sometimes we cry, or somewhere in between.

It was a little tricky finding the right entrance. The hospital had not updated their directions that they send in advance since renovating the building.

It felt weird being at a cancer center for migraines. There were people in the waiting room who were clearly suffering from cancer. Many of the cancer patients waiting for infusions and other treatments looked thin and weak.

I felt guilty. And I often feel guilty for my cancer journey (more on that later).

I thought: "Why does my infusion have to take place at a cancer center?" However, the people there showed me the reality of what cancer looks like for many.

Each of our stories is different. In fact, my cancer, chronic myeloid leukemia, is an invisible illness. You would never know I have cancer if you saw me walking along the street.

Happily, I heard a staff member tell one patient in the waiting room that this was to be his last treatment.

The staff member said, "Yeah, you'll follow up and see your doctor and go from there."

The patient had hope all over his face and a big smile. That moment made my day.

He wasn't expecting that exciting news. It's not the end of his journey, but that news gave him hope to keep going, I could only imagine.

Being in the waiting room reminded me of why I help cancer patients and survivors through Showing Up: Perspectives On Cancer, the global, weekly livestreamed show; this series of books and the in-person events we hold each year.

My why is to let other cancer patients, survivors and supporters know they are not alone and to encourage others to share their stories, when they are ready.

## My Story

I was originally diagnosed at age 28 in 2006 with chronic myeloid leukemia. I had discovered purple bruises on my leg. So, I went to my primary care physician. He took bloodwork and quickly called me to let me know I needed to go to the hospital right away. I immediately went with my parents and a family friend, who was so kind to drive us, to Westchester Medical Center in New York state.

While I was in the hospital for four days, I was diagnosed with chronic myeloid leukemia, a blood cancer. We do have a lot of cancer in our extended family – my grandparents, my uncles, aunts and more. My uncle had Hodgkins Disease, the only other blood cancer in the family of which I am aware.

I was surprised I had cancer – I don't know why because cancer is so prevalent in my family, but still, I was.

I have been very blessed during my cancer journey from a physical perspective. The only physical effects I have had allegedly are purple bruises on my leg when I was first diagnosed.

However, I did mention earlier that I've been struggling with severe migraines on and off for nine years, which is around the same time I have been taking the oral chemotherapy medication called Sprycel. Currently, I am temporarily not taking Sprycel to see if it may be the cause of the migraines.

I had some level of chronic myeloid leukemia for almost 15 years, when all of a sudden, my oncologist called one day to tell me I was cancer-free. He had done a genetic study, which measures how many leukemia cells you have in your body.

I stayed cancer-free for 1.5 years. I found out I was cancer free one month after launching the show "Showing Up: Perspectives On Cancer."

Hold on a second … I found out I was cancer free. Say, whattttt? I remember, that day I was so excited – it was such a relief. I remember telling my family and friends and feeling the excitement back from them as well.

But then I thought …

- What does this mean for how I want to live my life?
- How do I want to make more impact in the cancer community?
- How do I intentionally want to be happy?

Let me tell you, the hardest part of my specific cancer journey has been the mental and emotional effects:

- The inconsistency of it all.
- Being in cancer.
- Then out of cancer.
- Then in cancer.

As of January 2024, it is still with me. But that could change in a heartbeat.

Let me clarify that I've never had any physical effects during all of these changes in my cancer status.

But mentally and emotionally it's like, how do you live not knowing if you're going to be in cancer or out of cancer? And how much does it matter? Each situation is different, and each person's story is different.

Some things that I have done to help with my mental and emotional state are - identify what brings me peace.

For me, that's:

- Being in nature.
- Taking walks.
- Shooting photos and videos of nature.

And then sharing that on my social media. I get nice feedback from people about my photography and videos of the Delaware River in Northeast Pennsylvania. Also, of Raymondskill Falls just outside of Milford, Pa. That positive feedback feels good.

Granted, sometimes my mind does wander while I'm out in nature.

Sometimes that's a good thing, and sometimes I think too much about what's on my mind and heart.

I do encourage you to reflect:

- What are some things that currently make you happy?
- What are some things you want to do in the near future to make you happy?
- And then long-term — say 5 to 10 years out — what do you want to do then to make you happy?

Make a timeline along with your Happy List items.

So, for example, for me, nature currently brings me happiness. I try to get out in nature at least a few times a week (what I really want to do is schedule this time in my calendar, and I encourage you to schedule your happy time too, as though it were a business meeting).

Some things in 2023 I did to intentionally bring me happiness were going in a hot air balloon ride (it was so fricken' fun!) and going to the Macy's Thanksgiving Day Parade in New York City with my family. I hadn't been there since I was a child.

**(I encourage you to share in our Showing Up: Perspectives On Cancer Facebook Group, what are some things you intentionally want to do to bring you happiness?)**

Even in a cancer journey, it's important to find happiness.

In the short-term, I want to go sky-diving or hang-gliding. There are some weight requirements, so having these goals will make me focus on another goal I have – losing weight and improving my nutrition. This is something I've struggled with for some time.

I recently signed up for Weight Watchers (now called WW) to help me with this. What I love about Weight Watchers is you can eat anything in moderation.

In 2012 to 2013 I had lost 95 pounds, and I want to do that again.

In the long-term, I want to travel around the world. My happiness goals include continuing to make an impact in the cancer community – who knows what opportunities will open up in the next 5 to 10 years or what opportunities I will create?

Or what opportunities you will find or create.

But I do know that it is important for all of us to show up for ourselves (we are no good for anybody else if we don't take care of ourselves – I know this is easier said than done sometimes, but take one thing at a time).

For example, in 2023, I started seeing a therapist. I was having problems processing survivors' guilt, even though I know cancer isn't a competition.

Another challenge I had was figuring out how to communicate with the closest people in my life, especially expressing my wants and needs.

So, I now have a therapist. We've been meeting weekly for some time, and she helps guide me through hard conversations around cancer.

We each have our own perspectives.

As cancer patients.

Survivors.

And supporters.

It's important for us to listen to each other so we can learn from each other about our wants and needs.

Each patient, survivor and supporter has different needs, so it's not easy.

That is why it's so important that we communicate with each other, even when it's uncomfortable.

It's important also to show up for our family, friends and

colleagues who may also be struggling with cancer, even if we don't know what to say. The fact that they know we are there for them is the most important of all.

## The Story of Showing Up

When I started sharing my cancer story in June of 2021 after almost 15 years of having leukemia, I had no idea what would follow:

- More invitations to share my story — on blogs, on podcasts, live shows and virtual events. So grateful!
- Connecting with other cancer patients, survivors & supporters — sharing our stories one-on-one, in direct messages on Zoom calls and phone calls.
- And eventually launching the global, weekly livestreamed show "Showing Up: Perspectives On Cancer" — a safe space where cancer survivors and cancer supporters come together to share their stories and connect, as well as find resources that provide healing, hope and resilience. The shows are Wednesday at 8 pm EST.

My original show co-creator was Kara Oelker, then Erica Neubert Campbell and now Shannon Lee-Sin, who I met at Podfest Multimedia Expo in 2023.

So grateful for each of them, bringing their own unique perspectives and stories to the show.

Every week we have a conversation with a cancer patient, survivor or supporter. They share their stories & perspectives in our safe space livestreamed show, which is found on Facebook, LinkedIn, YouTube and Twitter.

The show started in November 2021, and on Wednesday Jan. 10, we celebrated our 100th episode by inviting you, our family, to join us on screen and share what Showing Up: Perspectives On Cancer means to you – how it has impacted you. We had giveaways and gave out awards.

The show has also led to the publication of the book "Perspectives On Cancer: Cancer Patients, Survivors & Supporters Share Their Stories" (Vol. 1) and now this one.

Also, we've held two in-person events as well, and the third is coming up Oct. 5 & 6, 2024 in Vermont (it will be so beautiful with the fall colors).

This show, the book, the event would not be happening without your support!!! So, thank you from the bottom of my heart.

And a special shout out goes to Joy Sohn, my wife, for helping out with this book, the in-person events and so much more!!!

In addition, another special shout out goes to Andrea Sanchez, my accountability partner for always encouraging me on all these crazy, impactful projects, to keep going, even when I haven't wanted to.

**In the Pages of This Book …**

you will find stories of healing, hope and resilience from cancer patients, survivors and supporters.

While reading these stories, there will be sad moments - you will need tissues (are you Team Puffs or Team Kleenex?), there will be silly moments, laughing moments, serious moments, happy moments – all the emotions.

But –

- You will learn from these authors;
- You will relate to pieces of their stories;
- You may find healing and inspiration;
- You will definitely find hope; and
- You may find that you want to connect to and reach out to the authors or myself.

Please feel free to reach out to us.

We are a community.

We are Showing Up.

# 2

# LOOSE KNEES: LEARNING TO RIDE THE WAVES AFTER CANCER

## BY SHANNON LEE-SIN

In Jamaica, we have always believed "prevention is better than cure." I've grown up my entire life hearing those words, but I never really understood what they meant until my own cancer diagnosis at 29 years of age.

I have had digestive issues since I was 17 years old, including chronic abdominal pain and intermittent blood in my stool. I reported my symptoms to my pediatrician and was diagnosed with a stomach ulcer, then prescribed antacids without any investigatory testing being performed.

In my high school Honors and AP Biology classes, I learned that blood in the stool is a sign of serious illness like colon cancer and it was typical in people over 50 years old. I brushed off my symptoms because in my mind I was too young for colon cancer.

After attending high school in Miami, I went to Jamaica to pursue my undergraduate studies in architecture. During that time, my symptoms got worse and more frequent. I sought medical attention but was constantly misdiagnosed, despite my symptoms being predominantly gastrointestinal in type, such as nausea, vomiting, abdominal pain and digestive issues such as constipation, diarrhea and blood in my stool.

Over the next four years, I was consistently misdiagnosed with bladder infections, hemorrhoids, gastroenteritis and reproductive issues such as ovarian cysts, endometriosis and polycystic ovarian syndrome, while I unknowingly had colorectal cancer growing within my body. I was seen by about 20 doctors, searching for answers, and unfortunately, they all misdiagnosed me without proper examinations and scans.

The nausea, pain and diarrhea were so intense that I went to the emergency room repeatedly. Since the beginning of this ordeal, I had been seen by internal medicine doctors, gynecologists, reproductive specialists, emergency room doctors and general practitioners but was never referred to a gastroenterologist.

I went to the emergency room repeatedly. People began to think my illness was all in my head, and so did I. I truly thought it was psychosomatic, although I felt there really was something seriously wrong. I wasn't a doctor, so what did I know? Culturally, I was taught not to question authority.

A week after completing my bachelor's degree, I traveled to Miami, in hopes of getting a diagnosis. No doctor would see me because I didn't have insurance, and I didn't qualify for Medicaid. The public clinic didn't have any appointments for at least four months. However, within a week of my arrival, my pain was so bad, I told my mom "I'd either have medical bills to pay, or she'd be paying for my funeral."

We went to the ER at Jackson South Community Hospital, where I underwent another ultrasound, where the doctors determined I had ovarian cysts and sent me home without admittance. Two days later, my mom came home from work and saw I was in severe pain, my abdomen was distended, and my skin had become orange in hue. We returned to the same ER, where I finally received my first CT scan along with blood work. I had a huge abscess in my abdomen, and I was in sepsis. I was treated with antibiotics and given a blood transfusion. The doctors said it was most likely a form of irritable bowel disease, colitis or diverticulitis. I spent five days recovering in the ICU.

The doctors wanted to treat the infection and inflammation in my colon to perform a colonoscopy, rather than perform invasive surgery.

However, the infection returned three times over the next four months, so on Oct. 4, 2011, I underwent emergency exploratory surgery. The surgery that was expected to take 45 minutes turned into a 10-hour ordeal. A week later, I was shocked with a diagnosis of Stage 3C colon cancer and becoming an ostomate.

I received my diagnosis more than a decade after I started experiencing symptoms as a teenager. It took me around 12 years from my first visit with my pediatrician in high school to get a diagnosis of Stage 3C colorectal cancer at 29. I want to be clear – my cancer, despite being late stage, did not appear in any of the scans I underwent.

I recovered in the hospital for four weeks. Just prior to being discharged, I was diagnosed with a pulmonary embolism. Within days of my discharge, I went to my first oncology appointment.

I read my pathology report prior to my first oncology appointment; I was empowered as a patient. I researched any term I did not understand in that report. I researched the typical treatments used and their side effects, what a carcinoembryonic antigen test was, and, of course, what my prognosis was.

I went into my first appointment empowered and armed with informed, educated questions. I was ready to make decisions, not have them made for me. I was determined to be an informed participant and not just a silent bystander.

Knowing the side effects of my chemotherapy and the fact that it increased my five-year survival rate from 50 percent to 75 percent made it a no-brainer to choose to undergo chemotherapy.

Despite the long-term effects, I would make that decision again in a heartbeat. Chemotherapy is what saved my life. Advocating for annual colonoscopies saved my life and keeps me cancer free.

My doctors have now agreed that I am at a low risk of a recurrence, but I am still high-risk for a new primary colorectal cancer because of my propensity for having polyps despite annual colono-scopies.

The weekend after my discharge, a month after my surgery and diagnosis, I attended my graduation ceremony in Jamaica that week-end. The following Monday, I returned to the United States to begin a rigorous six-month chemotherapy regimen, consisting of three continuous days of treatment bi-weekly. I struggled with getting back to "normal" even after treatment was completed.

Two weeks after my college graduation, my grandfather was diag-nosed with pancreatic cancer and passed away six weeks later. My grandfather was a steadfast male role model in my life. He taught me the importance of hard work, generosity, humility, faith and love. He was my grandmother's primary caregiver during her battle with Alzheimer's. I moved to Jamaica to take over her care, so my grandfa-ther could focus on loving her, without having to do the hard work in caring for her. My grandfather became my best friend, my biggest supporter and my biggest motivation in finishing my degree.

Watching my grandfather, my best friend, fight cancer and succumb to it was the hardest thing I have ever been through in my life. Watching a loved one fight cancer can be harder than having cancer itself. I endured both journeys simultaneously. The grief remains.

Fifteen months post-diagnosis, against my surgeon's recommen-dation, I had my ostomy reversal, because the ostomy negatively impacted my quality of life. That decision came with many chal-lenges. I have struggled with getting back to "normal," even after treatment was completed and over a decade after ostomy reversal.

After having a colostomy for 15 months, and while I was in the hospital recovering from my reversal surgery, I decided to pursue a Master of Architecture degree. I prepared my portfolio while in the hospital, and I delivered my application package to Florida International University three days after being released from the hospital, while still having over 60 staples in my abdomen from surgery.

I was offered the opportunity to work in England for a luxury residential design-build firm for the summer prior to starting school. However, two months before my first semester, as I was planning for my travels to England, a routine CT scan revealed lesions on my liver, suspicious of metastatic disease. This did not deter me; it actually emboldened me.

I went to England and came back to undergo biopsies and testing. As the friend who I was supposed to lodge with in England said, "whatever I had wouldn't kill me in two months." So, I took the once in a lifetime opportunity! Despite the unknown and undergoing constant routine testing and biopsies, I embarked on my studies and graduated in 2016. I knew I wanted a Master of Architecture whether I lived or died.

Life after cancer isn't easy. I am mentally, emotionally and physically exhausted. No one told me what my life would be like after treatment.

I still suffer from long-term side effects including PTSD, anxiety, depression, gastroparesis, chronic nausea, vomiting, diarrhea, neuropathy, chronic pain, chronic fatigue, liver damage, fertility issues and chemo brain – a not so funny way of saying I have cognitive dysfunction, not to mention the financial toxicity caused by my cancer diagnosis.

Colorectal cancer is preventable.

Treatable.

Beatable.

Self-advocacy has saved my life and continues to keep me alive. I have since become a fighter and advocate for others. I have advocated for annual colonoscopies for myself. I had 15 to 20 polyps in the 12 inches of colon removed during my surgery. I have never had a clean colonoscopy, and I've done at least one per year in my 12 years of survivorship.

I also advocate for others. I have shared my story in the *Miami Herald, On the Rise Magazine*, on the local news and in several webinars including Total Health, PBS and the Colon Cancer Foundation's Early Age Onset Colorectal Cancer Virtual Summit.

The fire of my advocacy is fueled by the fact that my story could have been like so many of my friends who I have lost. Their lives have been stolen. Their dreams have been stolen. Their futures have been stolen. Their potential has been stolen. They have been robbed of so much and so have their families. Little children have lost their mom or dad to this preventable disease.

Now children and teenagers are losing their lives to colorectal cancer as well. Mothers and fathers are burying their children. Brothers and sisters are grieving their siblings. I have a personal vendetta against colorectal cancer. I advocate fervently and passionately so there will be more stories of survival like mine. I'm 41 years old, a 12-year survivor and I am still well below the recently lowered recommended screening age of 45.

When I was diagnosed in 2011, being under the age of 50, I only had a one in 20 chance of having colorectal cancer. That same demographic, the under 45 population, is now at a one in five risk – that is 20 percent. The statistics have quadrupled in a little over a decade. In my time of survivorship, colorectal cancer has gone from the third cancer killer in this country and internationally to number two. By 2030, if trends continue, it will be the number one cancer killer in the world. This is a preventable disease.

Life after cancer can be quite difficult at times but not as bad as before diagnosis and during cancer treatment. However, there are also blessings. The purpose of life is to live with purpose. To enjoy and live every moment to the fullest. Also, to turn pain into passion and to be an advocate for others who are less aware and exposed to knowledge and resources.

As much as cancer has stolen from me, it has not killed my dreams. I have become an advocate for myself and others. I am learning to say goodbye to who I was. I no longer hold on to fear. I am no longer ashamed of my disease and the stigma it carries. I am no longer afraid to share my experiences to help others.

Despite cancer and its after-effects, I earned a Bachelor and a Master of Architecture and had a successful career in local government as a construction manager. I am near accomplishing accreditation as a Registered Architect.

I did all my advocacy work while working full-time. I used my free time and vacation time to continue my fight against colorectal cancer and make my own impact. Advocacy is my passion.

My advocacy brought me a new community and family. People who get me. People I can truly be my authentic self around. Something I've never had before. I found a safe place.

Cancer has made me fearless in many ways. It has made me value time. Time is the most inexpensive thing in the world, and also the most valuable, because it is something we don't ever get back. I focus on moments, memories, trying new things and going on adventures I never would have tried or done prior to my diagnosis. I try to get out and live every day!

Since cancer, I have become a paddleboarder and now a surfer – two things I never would have done. I am deathly scared of sharks, water I can't see in, alligators, crocodiles, snakes, rip tides and water deeper than my shoulders. I have overcome all my fears and journeyed out of my comfort zone. In doing so, what I used to fear has become my new comfort zone, as when I was surfing, I was so at peace out there in the ocean, I took a nap on my surfboard!

The first lesson you learn in surfing and paddleboarding is that the board is designed to float, or to ride the wave. We have to become one with the board in order to do the same. The trick in doing this is to keep loose knees.

This has been my mantra in life – to ride the waves of life with loose knees. Like in the ocean, it is easier to go with the current of life than fight against it.

This has transformed my life for 2023 and the ebbs and flows in life I encountered.

In November, due to continued discrimination, compounded with the long-term side effects from my cancer, including peripheral neuropathy and arthritis in my hip, I made the difficult decision to walk away from the career I risked my life for. I found my peace of mind, mental health and physical wellness were more important than a six-figure salary or title.

Since walking away from my career, I have decided to embrace being a full-time advocate in the war against colorectal cancer. I have never been more at peace or happier for as long as I can remember.

I have continuously stepped out of my comfort zone since making that decision. After finally taking the advice of my dear friend Lee Silverstein, colon cancer survivor and the former host of two successful podcasts – The Colon Cancer Podcast, which became the We Have Cancer Podcast, I have decided to enter the world of livestreaming. It only took about eight years of a 10-year friendship to get me to do this.

I launched my livestream, Blue Couch Chat, once I realized that Lee was on hospice. He was my first guest as planned, and unfortunately, he passed away five days after we livestreamed that episode.

I am now the co-host of a video podcast with Tim Sohn, Showing Up: Perspectives on Cancer, in which we interview people impacted by cancer in various ways. I have also been a featured guest on several video podcasts since then.

I have also officially launched my own YouTube livestream, Blue Couch Chat: The Safe Place to Talk About Your Sh!t. Like many, I have been isolated and excluded by my friends and family because of illness.

Culturally, as a Jamaican being of Asian and African descent, my other family members don't share their own cancer diagnoses or other health issues with other family members, and I am expected to handle my issues in the same manner. That is why I created a safe place for survivors to share their stories and find support. Every story is important and can help at least one other person.

As an abuse, sexual assault, domestic violence, suicide and cancer survivor, life has taught me many lessons. However, cancer has taught me the biggest lessons of all.

I have learned to love myself, fight for myself, be proud of me, be free to be me, step out of my comfort zone, to fully own my opportunities, to get out and thrive and to keep loose knees, while I ride the waves of life and enjoy the thrill of it all while that wave lifts me up and carries me on to bigger and better things!

Life is not just meant to be lived; it is intended to be enjoyed to the max.

# 3

# WHEN LIFE GIVES YOU LEMONS …
## BY AMANDA R. FERRARO

I was born with double pneumonia because at the time of my birth I had swallowed my mother's amniotic fluid. My first few days of life were spent in the NICU.

When I was a few months old I ended up contracting scarlet fever and again was hospitalized. At the age of 7, my maternal aunt was diagnosed with Ewing Sarcoma, a form of lung cancer. That was the first time in my life I heard the word cancer.

Throughout my aunt's cancer journey I witnessed my aunt lose her hair, be very sick and fight for her life. Even though I was only 7 years old, my family was very open and honest about what cancer was, what it meant and how together as a family we were going to combat it.

I remember my mom changing my aunt's dressings for her pick line. I got to see the community rally around my aunt, sending her donations and flowers, showing so much love and support to her. I remember going to doctors' visits, asking questions and genuinely learning about what my aunt was going through.

For a child, that can be a lot to take in, but luckily my family is so amazing. They were able to explain to me in a way that made me feel proud of my aunt. No matter where we went, my aunt had a smile on her face. She never let cancer take over her humility or humor.

Cancer didn't define who she was, and she never let it take over her life, even though it tried. Being a witness to how strong my aunt was really made an imprint on me, and I believe that I learned how to advocate for myself through what I was able to witness.

A few months after my aunt was diagnosed with cancer, I ended up having my very first brain surgery. I was having headaches, and I was very sensitive to noise. Loud noises would really scare me, and I was having trouble in school.

My parents ended up taking me to Children's Hospital of Philadelphia where the neurosurgeon saw that there was an arachnoid cyst on my cerebellum. The next day I was prepped for brain surgery. A stent was placed to drain the hydrocephalus, which is excessive cerebral spinal fluid in the brain, and it seemed to cure all my symptoms.

I was very lucky to have parents who advocated for me. My pediatrician at the time called me a hypochondriac and told my parents I was complaining to get attention, but because I was so persistent about how I was feeling, they knew something was wrong. This was the first time that I learned that I had to advocate for myself.

A few months after I had my first brain surgery, my grandfather passed away. This was the very first time I had dealt with death, and it was very difficult for me. I didn't understand why he was taken away from me, but I knew that expressing how I felt made me feel good. It made me feel like I was able to take a deep breath.

A year after my first brain surgery, my younger sister Samantha was diagnosed with brain cancer. My mom had brought my sister with her to an appointment with my aunt's oncologist, who suggested that they go to Children's Hospital of Philadelphia. With my history of having a cyst on the brain, he knew that it would be a good idea to seek expert medical advice. My sister was diagnosed with Primitive Neuroectodermal Tumor.

Because of my sister's cancer, my family dynamic changed quite drastically.

My mother stayed at the hospital with my little sister who was undergoing chemotherapy and radiation. My father stayed at our house and went to work every day so he could keep the insurance, so my sister was able to go through treatment. I lived with my grandmother.

It was during this time that I first started writing journals. I was going through a lot of emotions between feeling abandoned and angry. I was missing my parents, and I was afraid that my sister was going to die. That's a lot for a 10-year-old.

My parents decided to put me through therapy, but I found comfort in writing down what I was feeling. Writing benefited me more. To me, writing was a way for me to release my emotions, and it helped loosen the burden of dealing with reality.

Luckily, my sister went into remission, and we were able to get our life back on track. Once my sister and my aunt were both cancer free, our lives returned to "normal." I played softball, soccer, piano and participated in cheerleading. I also loved writing short stories and journaling.

When my paternal grandfather passed away, I reverted to journaling my feelings to let go of the hurt and the emptiness that I felt. For 10 years, I went through life learning that journaling my feelings really helped me. Although I wasn't the best language arts student, I felt that writing was an outlet for me.

When I was a senior in high school, I started to have bad headaches again, but doctors couldn't find anything wrong and called me a hypochondriac again. All the tests that had been done were normal, so my parents took me back to Children's Hospital of Philadelphia to see if they could figure out what was going on with me.

I'll never forget the neurosurgeon looking at me and saying, "If you're lying, you need to stop, and if you're telling the truth, I will do exploratory brain surgery to find out what's going on, but it's up to you."

I mean, imagine the weight that I felt on my shoulders at that time. On our way home from that doctor's visit, I told my parents to call them back and make the appointment for the brain surgery because I knew something was wrong with me. It was at that moment that I learned no one understood what I was going through, and I was the only one who could express what I was going through.

My parents called the brain surgeon back and scheduled the appointment for surgery. When the doctor cut my skull open, my cyst was so big that it had ruptured, causing me to lose two pints of blood. When he tried to tie the cyst into the fourth ventricle, he ended up nicking one of the nerves to my eyes, which caused me to end up completely cross-eyed after surgery. When the neurosurgeon came in for my post-op visit, he looked at me and said, "you were right." That changed my life!

About six months after having surgery, I started having headaches again. The neurosurgeon at Children's Hospital of Philadelphia referred me to another neurosurgeon in New York's Mount Sinai Hospital because of my age.

In 2007, I had my third brain surgery to put a complete ventriculoperitoneal (VP) shunt placed into my brain, down through my stomach to relieve some of the hydrocephalus that was causing me to have headaches. Unfortunately, because I had grown up with so much pressure in my brain when the shunt was placed, my body could not function without some pressure. So, a month after having my third brain surgery, I had a fourth to put a programmable valve in. I was very happy with the surgery and proud of myself for advocating my needs.

After the recovery process, I was able to start college and find a job. I thought that my life was on track, and I never could have imagined needing a fifth brain surgery.

However, three years after having the VP shunt placed, I started having the very same symptoms all over again.

I ended up going to several doctors who could not find anything wrong with me and told my parents once again that it was all in my head and I was doing this for attention. Luckily, I had an amazing primary care physician who knew that I wasn't a hypochondriac. He believed me and put so much effort into finding out what was going on.

He ended up sending my medical records to the chief neurosurgeon at Johns Hopkins University Medical Center and got me an appointment. Because all the tests prior came back negative, the neurosurgeon decided to do one last nuclear medicine test. The test showed that I was right and that there was a blockage of some sort in this VP shunt.

Again, because I advocated for myself, and I knew that something was going on with my body, I needed another brain surgery. In 2011, I went under the knife. My old VP shunt was taken out, and a new ventriculoarterial (VA) shunt placed. After the surgery, as protocol, my neurosurgeon sent my old shunt to infectious disease.

After testing, they came into my hospital room fully dressed in head-to-toe gear and explained to my parents and I that I had a staph infection in my shunt, and if it had gone to my brain, I could have died. No one would have known why.

That is when I realized speaking up and advocating could save lives. Since the infection could be deadly, I needed to stay in the hospital for an additional two weeks and receive around-the-clock antibiotics via intravenous line. I couldn't believe that I was right again, and I was so thankful that my primary care physician listened to me. If he hadn't, I wouldn't be here today.

After recovering from my sixth brain surgery, life was great. I ended up meeting the man of my dreams, and in 2013 I got pregnant with my son. When I was 10 weeks pregnant, I started having some problems with my heart, and an ultrasound showed that my shunt was scraping the right atrium of my heart.

At 16 weeks pregnant, I ended up needing my seventh brain surgery. The neurosurgeon had to shorten my VA shunt so it wouldn't penetrate my heart. My son was monitored the whole surgery, and on Dec. 24, 2013, I delivered a healthy baby boy.

Being a mother was an absolute dream. I was so happy. I stopped at nothing to make sure that my son had everything he ever needed or could want. I could never have imagined life without him. For three years of his life, I was by his side 24/7, until May 15 of 2017.

I went to the emergency room one night because I was having

trouble breathing. I was very fatigued, and I felt like something was wrong with my heart. I could barely walk from my car to the emergency room doors. After speaking with the physician on call, he ended up doing blood work and looked into my records to see what he could find.

At a previous ER visit, just two months prior, test results showed there were 15 blast cells in my blood. Once the ER doctor had viewed all of my chart information and read over the new blood tests, he came into my room, pulled up a chair, sat down and told me that I was going to need a consultation with an oncologist. He was going to prep me to get a blood transfusion because my hemoglobin was so low that if I had fallen asleep that night, I could have died.

The next day when the oncologist came into the hospital room, he nonchalantly stood there and told me that I had leukemia and that they were going to prepare me for chemotherapy because it was "bad." He had no bedside manner and didn't even acknowledge the fact that I was hysterical.

My very first phone call was to my mom letting her know what the doctor had said and telling her that I needed her ASAP. The second call was to my boyfriend's mom because I didn't know how to break the news that I had cancer. I just couldn't bear giving him the news.

We ended up wanting to get a second opinion, and I was moved to Robert Wood Johnson at the Rutgers National Cancer Institute of New Jersey. The hospital staff there specialized in acute myeloid leukemia, which was my diagnosis, and I knew I was in good hands.

On May 17, 2017, I started my first induction chemotherapy. The days were long and hard. I would receive phone calls from my son where he would be crying and begging me to come home. He was only 3 1/2 at the time and didn't understand why I wasn't there. He thought maybe that he was being bad and that is why I had left. It was the hardest part of being diagnosed with cancer.

Thankfully, I had amazing doctors and hospital staff who listened to my needs. I knew this would be one of the hardest things I would ever go through, and although I did not want to be there, I knew that

I had to fight for my life so I could be the mother I always wanted to be.

With each blood draw or test that was done, I made sure that I got the results, and I put them in a binder. A week after starting chemotherapy, I needed an emergency appendectomy because my appendix almost ruptured. It felt like my world was crumbling down around me and there was nothing I could do about it. However, 33 days after receiving the worst diagnosis of my life, I was able to go home and hug my son.

I was told I was in remission on Valentine's Day of 2018, and that was one of the very best days.

In my mind, life was going to go back to the way it was, so I started making plans of what I wanted to do to make up for the time we had lost. It was hard at first for my son to accept me though. The feeling of abandonment was a burden on his heart. We ended up putting my son into play therapy, which was one of the best decisions of my life because it truly helped him to express what he was feeling.

Because of my love for journaling, I ended up starting a Facebook page for my family so they could stay updated on what I was going through. I used that page as a diary of sorts. Although I was seeing a therapist, for me, writing was therapy. It was a way to let go of all the negative energy I was holding on to. I posted everything from the ambulance ride to the hospital to my mom shaving my head. I was open and honest, and I didn't hold anything back. It truly helped me get through each day.

Seven months after learning I was cancer free, I ended up relapsing, and because I had been through my first cancer journey, I knew what I was in for, or so I thought. When the cancer came back, my oncologist gave me a 10 percent chance of living because of a genetic mutation.

I ended up needing to have a stem cell transplant to save my life. I was very open and honest throughout my whole cancer journey and through my blog, I started connecting with so many other cancer patients who were in my situation. I learned that I was not alone in what I was going through. I learned that by advocating for myself and sharing my experience I was able to connect and help others feel like they were not alone.

A fire was lit in my heart once I realized that by sharing my story, I could help other people. I became determined to share my story in hopes of making change for others within the world of cancer, not just for patients of blood cancer, but for all cancer patients. Patients who have children or are low income. Patients that feel they have no voice or feel alone in their journey. What I have been through in my life and how I learned to advocate for myself became a passion to advocate for others.

I started a website, www.cancerisanasshole.com, so I could help patients and their families find resources that they were so desperately needing. I started writing blogs and articles so others could read what it is like to have cancer and how to help family members go through their cancer journey.

I wanted people to understand what it was like to get life-changing news, and I wanted them to understand the anxiety and PTSD that cancer patients and survivors go through. I want to make cancer a topic of discussion and not a taboo word. I want to make a change.

I have been lucky enough to share my story through a TEDx Talk, a publication in a medical journal, several articles with different cancer magazines, podcasts and fundraisers through the Leukemia & Lymphoma Society. However, my work is not done.

My goal is to become a board-certified patient advocate so I can work with governments and hospitals to make the lives of cancer patients a little bit easier, and through my work with the National Coalition for Cancer Survivorship, create a survivorship checklist for all cancer patients for post treatment care needs.

Although no one knows what the future holds, I know mine is bright, however long that may be. With God by my side, faith in my heart, family and friends supporting me, Jesse (my love) and Isaac's (my son) love, I know that I will be able to achieve whatever I put my mind to. I have been through hell and back, but I feel it was for a reason. One I may never know, but that won't stop me.

# 4

# FROM WEDDING VOWS TO MEDICAL DIAGNOSIS: OUR YEARS NAVIGATING CANCER AS NEWLYWEDS

## BY JOE TOWER AND ANNA TOWER-KÖVESDI

"Are you sure you want to do this with me?" she asked through tears in the exam room when the nurses had left. "Don't even ask me that," he replied, eyes red from crying and fatigue.

We were waiting for confirmation from the ER team at Mercy Regional Medical Center in Durango, Colo., about air transport north to Denver, after being told about Anna's wildly concerning blood numbers. It was December, a week before Christmas – our first as a married couple after our wedding that summer.

"There's a 90 percent chance it's leukemia," the doctor said. "What's the other 10 percent?" Anna had asked, to which the doctor just shook her head.

A cancer diagnosis can be the most challenging news a person (or persons) can ever receive. For any couple, facing a life-threatening illness together can seem like an impossibility; it will put every one of your collective strengths to the test. For us, after a short marriage, and not even a year living together in the same country, the concept was a tragic and drastic turn.

We first crossed paths working for the same international startup. Joe was based out of the U.S. – Los Angeles – and Anna from

Budapest, Hungary, at the company's home office. It was a love story that started in project management, with Anna booking travel for Joe to meet a deadline. On LinkedIn, innocent flirting blossomed into a full-blown across-the-world office romance.

Initially, managing a long-distance relationship – 6,000 miles and an eight-hour time difference – was intensified with the compounded challenges of COVID, quarantine, border restrictions, paperwork and immigration. It all seemed like life was putting our relationship to the ultimate test. But after finally being granted a visa for Anna to move to the U.S. so we could wed, it was only a brief respite before we realized that our greatest tests were yet to come.

So, only five months after we got married – after a brief bout of coronavirus and then holiday trips to Florida and Chicago – Anna began exhibiting what we now know to be textbook symptoms of blood cancer. A few days later we were in the ER, late into the night, and we first heard about sub-type Acute Lymphoblastic Leukemia (ALL). Late that night, she was airlifted to Denver for formal diagnosis and immediate treatment. Our lives were never the same.

Though mysterious symptoms had given us pause – fatigue, breathlessness, bruises – the nightmare really began with a phone call.

"...pack a bag, bring your husband, be here within an hour," the ER supervisor told Anna on a Sunday night at 9.

We'd spent the day at urgent care, addressing her general feeling of unwellness. The general consensus was that it could be attributed to some anemia or perhaps even long COVID. What we know now is that her leukemia had decimated her bone marrow.

She was days away from a stroke, or under the right circumstances, one wrong move away from a bleed. It was an interminable drive on dark county roads, made in fraught silence, before we arrived at the ER to get that unforgettable news: "There's a 90 percent chance it's leukemia."

With Anna set to make the cold and terrifying flight to Denver alone, Joe faced another challenge – Driving back to the home we'd only just established together, to pack their bags for Denver and leave everything they'd known up to that point overnight – unplanned, unprepared, in shock.

This alone would have been enough. But over the next few days, from Presbyterian St. Luke's Hospital in Denver, we received Anna's formal diagnosis of B-cell Acute Lymphoblastic Leukemia Ph negative, and learned that while it's highly treatable, it demands an extended treatment – three years – setting us on yet another new course, facing new challenges, both expected and unforeseen.

Fortunately, at this moment, we feel safe to say that Anna's done with a nearly two-year treatment, maintaining extended remission.

It has been 655 days since the diagnosis, and more than 60 of them spent inpatient, plus countless hours in the clinic, getting chemo infusions, blood transfusions, bone marrow biopsies, lab draws, lumbar punctures, blood thinner injections, high-dose steroids, antiviral tablets, antibiotics, sedatives, port insertion and removal surgeries, plus pokes, prods, tests, trials, X-rays, ECGs and EKGs.

But the true challenges have not been in those big numbers. The real challenges have been in our day-to-day. When our journey together took this sharp turn, we decided that it was no longer about building a life but declaring that it wouldn't be the end.

That was a lesson we would have to learn again and again.

Six months into treatment, just as she was gearing up to a "maintenance phase," a stomach infection led to 10 days in the hospital. She lost fifteen pounds, became dehydrated, was in and out of consciousness and required a wheelchair to move.

Weeks later, during what was supposed to be a routine blood draw, our oncologist told us that a recent bone marrow biopsy result showed signs that a secondary blood cancer had reared its head. In an attempt to evade targeted chemotherapy, her ALL had mutated into Acute Myeloblastic Leukemia (AML). Unusual, but not impossible, he scheduled Anna for immediate admission to the hospital for a 28-day chemotherapy induction phase to get her back to remission, along with prep for a bone marrow transplant.

All over again, we re-lived the diagnosis. We were scared and desperate, like the better part of a year we'd already spent powering through was for nothing.

So, after lots of tears and tantrums, some meditation and mindset, we had gotten ourselves ready to face everything again: a significant round of chemotherapy and the trial and trauma of a bone marrow transplant.

But then, mere hours before a scheduled infusion, the oncologist returned, glanced at Joe, then Anna, and knelt at the foot of the bed. He informed us that the results from a follow-up biopsy looked more promising than previously.

He proposed delaying chemo, pending more detailed results. The following day, more encouraging news led to Anna's discharge, though still no certainty. There was only a plan to observe and report how Anna's body would respond on its own – was her marrow producing rogue cancer cells or simply recovering from months of chemotherapy and coming back to life?

Following this break from chemo, during which we were able to take a shared sigh of relief, and after which Anna's AML was declared a misdiagnosis, we resumed her treatment schedule. This subsequent phase would be the final but most protracted segment of the protocol: daily oral chemo, monthly IV chemo, steroids, weekly clinic, and frequent lumbar punctures comprised the routine for the next two years.

A few weeks into this phase, fatigued from the toll of a year of chemo, an infection and a diagnosis scare, another appointment with our oncologist produced an unexpected new turn.

He presented various options for the path forward. Anna was given a choice to complete the treatment as planned, enduring a two-year maintenance phase or opt for a new treatment – the 2014 FDA-approved immunotherapy Blincyto, specifically designed for Anna's leukemia subtype. He expressed reservations about subjecting Anna to so much more chemo, given her remission status and citing its toxicity and associated risks. While neither option offered a significantly lessened susceptibility for relapse, with the immunotherapy, there was a potential for milder side effects and less permanent bodily damage existed.

The Blincyto treatment entailed cycles of a 28-day, 24/7 infusion with Anna connected to an IV all day, every day for almost a month.

An IV is accessed via a chest port, and the portable infusion pump is carried by the patient continuously for four weeks. Then there are two weeks off infusion at the culmination of each cycle. At the onset of the first three cycles, another hospital stay was required – once again bringing with it lots of needles, IV lines and initial treatment symptoms of high fever, muscle aches and lingering fatigue. The plan for Anna was to complete six months of Blincyto cycles, with the potential that she might continue for another six months. On the flip side, after the first six months, if her marrow samples looked good, Anna could potentially be finished with treatment.

After thoroughly discussing all perspectives, Anna opted for immunotherapy.

The prospect that the treatment could conclude almost a year earlier than planned was both unbelievable and hopeful, and the idea of a significantly shorter treatment duration became an anchor for our will to press on – and with it, perhaps at first, the promise of a "return" to a "normal" life. While a year may seem insignificant in the grand scheme of things, during the rigors of a cancer journey, it can mean, quite literally, everything.

An initially planned four or five cycles of Blincyto quickly expanded to a total of six, translating to nine months tethered to infusion, a needle in Anna's chest. Yet, throughout the nine months, with an end to treatment on the horizon, we had been trying desperately to embrace life – we moved up near Boulder, we built a new home, explored our new town, restaurants, hiking trails, the movie theater; we adopted a puppy; we returned to full-time work.

There was an absence of hours devoted to the illness, with fewer side effects and less scheduled clinic visits. With it came more hours filled with the usual challenges of "normal" life – the garage needs to be organized, the dog is acting like a nut, there's grocery shopping to be done.

Just like those difficult day-to-day trials of our cancer journey, it became clear that we did not have the skills to cope with them. Suddenly, we found ourselves having to adapt all over again, which is when a lingering question surfaced: when will our life ever go back to normal?

We don't talk about much because the ramifications and effects of cancer are so varied and encompass such a broad range of trauma and tragedy. But the common perception is that the expulsion of a particular cancer from the body and the end of its harrowing treatment bring with it an immediate sense of relief, joy, happiness, an easy return to normal. Perhaps it's as if cancer hadn't ever happened at all.

But it isn't true. Life is never the same again, and the day-to-day challenges when the journey is over is only the start to a new journey.

Oftentimes, while the patient becomes a survivor, drawing strength from this new identity, the caregiver can lose their identity and be left with a sense of emptiness. For patients and their support systems, the transition into the aftermath of the experience can create rifts.

In addition to the exhaustion both mentally and physically, couples like us – newer ones who didn't have an established foundation to the relationship going into the experience, but drew strength from it – can feel the sense of "starting over."

Although embracing gratitude and appreciating the small things does become a new norm as you make your way through a cancer journey, implementing that new ethos when you're re-confronted with real life can sometimes be harder than it sounds.

Rebuilding oneself is essential, both individually and as a couple. We are both in search of meaning in life and how we want to live it. This goes for our lives independently and our life together. One must constantly try to rediscover oneself, determine what the "new" normal is, contemplate their needs and wants, decide how one wants to act and discern what is truly important.

During the treatment, roles shifted instantly to patient and caregiver, and our roles of husband and wife, man and woman, were lost – they often are. We find ourselves in the position of having to start constructing our lives together again, despite all of the adversity we'd already endured just to get started the first time.

It's just six weeks since the end of treatment for Anna's cancer, and we're aware it's still new. It's also a point in the journey we were never fully confident we'd reach. But it's still surprising for us to grapple with these surreal feelings – uncertainty, frustration, impatience. Feelings we didn't think we would encounter at this point. Where do we begin? What can we do to make up for lost time? How do we proceed? We find ourselves desperately seeking answers, but perhaps we're still formulating the questions in the first place.

One thing is certain for us though: just when you think the journey is over, you have to start learning how to do everything – life included – again.

We are thankful to have been able to navigate this journey together so closely, acknowledging that our shared experience has only made us stronger. Our focus is on the lessons learned, the wisdom gained and the cherished relationships in our lives.

Our heartfelt gratitude extends to Presbyterian St. Luke's Medical Center, the Colorado Blood Cancer Institute, Dr. Marcello Rotta and Blair McKown.

# 5

# WHEN WE LOSE THE BEST

## BY DR. ASHOK BHATTACHARYA

"What's wrong mummy?" "Nothing. Don't forget to wear a warm sweater; it's cold outside."

That was my mother – hiding her problems and worrying about mine. I soon found out it was cancer. She had Peau d'orange. It's a late finding in breast cancer where the skin is dimpled like an orange. She hid it for too long. At the time of diagnosis, she had breast cancer cells swarming through her blood stream looking for places in her body to attack.

She was only 44. I was 18.

My mother was born in London, England, in 1934. She watched the Battle of Britain in 1940 from a bed in a hospital situated on a hill far away from London. She had rheumatic fever, which affected her heart, and in those days prolonged bed rest was the only treatment. The beds had itchy wool blankets, which made her squeamish for the rest of her life.

She entered art college where she met my father in 1956. My father was a charismatic, idealist who left India to get away from his famous family and study medicine in London. India became independent from Britain in 1947, and many young Indian men came to the United Kingdom looking to build a new life. My father was likely suffering from burnout and took art classes as a therapy. That's where they met.

Soon after, they were married, and three pregnancies later, they had five children. Yes, my mother had two sets of twins with four kids under 2 years old.

If you haven't guessed yet, I am the middle child and a classic one: hard done by, I never pushed to the front of the line, hypersensitive, empathic to a fault and always feeling that life is unfair.

I've always felt responsible for others.

As children we were subject to racism. The British didn't like the 'half-breeds' coming into their school systems; my twin and I were deemed "retarded." My parents decided not to stay, and we came to Newfoundland, Canada, in 1968. My father worked as a psychiatrist in a huge hospital and my mother became one of Canada's first art therapists at the same hospital.

That's where it happened, at least that's what I think. When I visited her at work, the smells were so strong. She had lots of carcinogenic oil paints and cleaners in her little room with poor ventilation. She didn't wear rubber gloves, and I've always wondered if that continuous exposure jeopardized her health.

Newfoundland was good to us. My father was a human rights activist, and my siblings and I were frequently in the newspaper winning awards and competitions. Ironically, Bhattacharya became a well known name in Newfoundland.

My mother and I were very close. I don't remember her ever saying she loved me. I knew she did. She was more like a friend than a mom. She was prone to fits of temper. She was stuck with her five children while my father was at the hospital doing night shifts. With six strong personalities around me, I became the quiet one. My mother was stoic but child-like in some ways. I always felt I had to protect her.

Home life was full of drama, not the good kind. Things began to fall apart when I was 15 years old. I could see my parents drifting apart. Then the cancer came.

My mother underwent a radical mastectomy. The "stiff upper lip" survivor of World War II had to face a new war inside her body. The only time I saw my mother cry was when she found out her father had died. She motioned for me to leave her alone as she read the telegram from England. I wanted to hug her; I was confused by her reaction and let her grieve alone.

The cancer changed my mother. Her personality changed. She became more outgoing; she developed a sense of humour and loved a dirty joke. She also started standing up to my father and created her own social connections. Their marriage couldn't take it. I was stuck trying to look after my mother and father while trying to keep the family functioning, but now our family had cancer.

My siblings reacted differently. I felt like an only child in a crowd with no one to share my feelings with. "You're too sensitive" was the usual response I got. My mother and I got tighter during that time. When I was 19, I found out I was accepted to medical school where I would soon learn of the disease, treatment and prognosis of my mother's condition. The more I learned, the more I realized she was going to die; I just didn't know when. Please don't feel too sad as you read this; there were lots of beautiful moments. We went out to shows, saw movies, went to restaurants and laughed a lot. Every moment became precious.

In September 1980 I started med school, and my parents divorced. I had to hide. I was playing in a semi-professional rock band, living in a bad area of town and pretending everything was fine. I was terrified that the medical school might discover my circumstances, and I worried that I would be kicked out. I was starring in an Academy Award-winning performance of my surreal life. I still feel shame about this.

After her mastectomy, my mother got five years before the cancer declared war on her pleura —the shiny lining between her lungs and her chest wall. She underwent an excruciating procedure to burn her lungs to her inner chest wall. I felt so helpless to do anything that would soothe her pain. I knew this was the beginning of the end.

My mother was a beautiful and vibrant woman — Helen Mirren reminds me of my mom. The mastectomy left my mother's arm twice the size of the other as the lymphatic drainage was blocked when the armpit nodes were removal. It didn't slow her down. She volunteered at the hospital to support women newly diagnosed with breast cancer. She looked like the role model of health and championed the idea that "cancer can be beaten." She was inspirational to many women. I was so proud of her.

After my parents' divorce, I felt even more responsible for my mother. I went to her medical appointments and helped her with the insensitive insurance forms. Even when she was dying, the forms still asked, "expected date of return to work." All I could do was be there for her. I told her that all the time.

By my final year of medical school, I didn't have the money to fly to Toronto do an in-person interview for the internship match, and I stayed in Newfoundland for my internship year — July 1984 to June 1985. My mother and I lived together. It was a beautiful time. We morphed from son and mother into best friends. We shared a year when her cancer was quiet.

By July 1985, I relocated to Toronto, Ontario, to start my training in psychiatry. It was a dream come true for me. Within a year my mother also moved to Ontario; she met the man she would soon marry. For a while, my mother seemed happy, calm and grounded. I even helped them build a beautiful home from the ground up on a lovely piece of land. I'm not handy — yes, I actually broke a hammer while hitting a nail. (Who does that?)

One evening, my mother and I were in a roadhouse restaurant — the ones that have butcher paper on the tables and a cup of wax crayons. I ripped off a little piece of the brown paper, wrote a little note with a pen and gave it to my mother while we drew silly pictures on the table with the crayons. I was scared for my mother's health, but I had to be optimistic and reflect that to her.

My best friend, Niels, was doing his Ph.D. in Trinidad. I decided it would be a good idea to visit him. We were two young bachelors, and I thought we would have some "fun on the beach." It was April 1986, and it was low season for tourism. Instead of finding the company of others, we deepened our relationship; we spent all our time talking and sharing ideas about life.

One memory stands out. We were sitting on the warm sand — just the two of us — on an expansive beach while the huge red sun was disappearing behind the horizon. The ocean was orange and placid. The only disruption was the silver glimmer of hundreds of flying fish leaping out of the water to catch flies. It was a perfect moment. I also saw Halley's Comet as it toured its 76-year orbit around earth. It was one of many signs.

It was only a few months later, while performing best man duties at my twin brother's wedding, that I met the woman I would marry. My wife is the kind of person who puts everyone else first before herself. My mother took an instant liking to her, and it was my mother who told me about a sale on diamonds. It was her way of encouraging me to propose. We married on Nov. 11, 1987.

The cancer cold war in my mother's body erupted, and the cease fire was over. The peritoneum, the lining inside her abdomen, was seeded by cancer that exuded a thick greenish cancerous sludge. It had to be removed by inserting a tube to drain it. My wife was a tremendous support to my mom, accompanying her at all those painful procedures.

Within my mother's belly was a tumor that would become a hardened mass the size of a volleyball. Because she was young-looking, people mistook her for pregnant. Palliative chemotherapy took her beautiful hair. We had our first child, and all the pictures from that time show a healthy little baby held by a fragile facsimile of my mother, struggling to keep a smile on her face. She was in unbearable pain.

My mother and her husband decided to move back to Newfoundland as she wanted to be by the ocean. It was difficult for me. In those days there was no FaceTime, only phone calls. She was getting sicker, and the palliative measures weren't controlling her pain. My wife and I had our daughter in March 1990.

It was getting hard to fly back and forth from Toronto to St. John's,

Newfoundland, with any regularity. I could feel my mother letting go. She has always focused on an upcoming event: a graduation, a birth, a wedding, Christmas, and the visits we could arrange. The time she had left was getting shorter, and she knew it. "I'm too young to die," she said with her pleading green eyes piercing my soul. She was so scared.

It was a cool November day in Ontario when the call came. "You need to get on a plane right now." The next day, I was with my siblings around the hospital bed where my mother was lying motionless. She was going in an out of consciousness as the doctors had her on heavy doses of morphine in an effort to 'make her comfortable.'

There was a brief moment in those few days when she woke up and was quite lucid. She made predictions that later came true. My mother never really accepted her death. The cancer made that decision for her. Her husband was beside himself and was the last of us to say, "It's OK if you need to go."

I was sleeping in the hospice adjacent to the hospital on Saturday morning, Nov. 10, 1990, at 8:30 a.m. when the nurse called my room. I ran over to where my mother was. She was gone. Her withered body didn't look like her. The sparkle in her eyes wasn't there anymore. Her grey hand was gnarled and claw-like. I kissed her forehead and said goodbye. She was only 56 years old.

As I was the executor of her will, I was going through some of her personal things, including her purse. After emptying it, I saw a little piece of paper in the corner. I took it out and unfolded it. I recognized it; it was the piece of butcher paper I had given her at the restaurant 2 years earlier. It read: "I will always look after you."

## My Friend, Niels

I met Niels in grade school in St. John's, Newfoundland, in September 1968. We had both just arrived from England, our fathers were psychiatrists of Indian descent, and my mother was British, and Neil's mother, Ursula, was German. Ursula was my first 'friend's mom crush.'

Neils and I were inseparable until our university years when our education plans diverted. I started medical school, and Neils pursued a Ph.D. in anthropology. I have two brothers, but Niels was my soul brother. We told each other things that were never uttered to anyone else. Our relationship went beyond friendship; we were connected on a different level.

Niels was scrupulous about his health: ate well, never smoked, was a light social drinker, exercised and took tons of vitamins. I think that's what did it, the vitamins. He was always scared of cancer. Longevity ran in his family with family members living into the 90s.

"Niels, I'm here. I can hop on a train and be in Oxford in a few hours."

"Sorry man, I just don't want to get COVID."

"I understand. I'll just wave up at your window from the street."

"Naah, that's OK. Spend time with your grandson; I'll be fine."

"OK, but if you change your mind, I'll be there."

"Thanks man..."

On the plane home to Toronto, I knew I would never see him again. We'd known each other for 53 years. It's the deepest and longest relationship I've ever had or will ever have. If a relationship can be measured by time and depth, Niels was that person for me.

He died a week later on Oct. 16, 2021.

A few days later, I wrote a song and made a video for Niels. His wife called and asked if I could write a song for his eulogy. I told her it was already done. She played it at his virtual funeral. I can't watch it without crying.

Niels lives in my heart now, next to my mother and many other dear people I have lost over the years. The loss of Niels feels heavy, numbing, and I still cry, especially if a song he liked comes on the radio.

My wife and I were able to fly to England — after meeting my daughter's new son — in April 2023. We arranged a side trip to Oxford where Niels's wife happily hosted us. She was still deep in grief and hadn't ventured out much. We took her out to a nearby pub, and she said it was the first time she had been out since Niels had been sick. She was smiling with a real smile. This would have made Niels happy.

I had a rental car; we were able to go to the cemetery where Niels was resting. It was a beautiful spring day. I knelt down beside his grave.

*"I love you Niels. I'm here now. I know you had to go, and you are in my heart...we will meet again my friend."*

I have learned so much from my cancer journeys with so many people — some friends, some family, some patients, all amazing humans who left my life too soon. I really only have two words when offering support to someone with cancer: SHOW UP.

# 6

# FIERCE, FABULOUS & FLAT
## BY BRANWYN LEE

Everyone diagnosed with breast cancer quickly learns that his or her journey is unique. You will meet people along the way with similarities - maybe it's cancer in the same breast, same chemo cocktail, cancer spreading to the lymph nodes, etc... There are many choices we each will have to make, and those decisions are the best for us and only us. For me, the only thing I was certain about from the second I learned I had breast cancer was: I want these breasts GONE; I want to be flat.

Hearing the words "you have cancer" was something that I never thought I would hear. Yes - there was always that possibility, something that you think about when you learn that a family member is battling, a friend, a co-worker, a child. However, I truly never thought I'd be the one hearing I have breast cancer.

Why? Maybe because I was young (39), in shape, always took my preventive care seriously, even had done genetic testing three months prior, showing no markers for 47 types of cancers and BRAC negative.

So, why am I getting this call telling me otherwise?

I was unable to formulate any other words other than "what do you mean?" only to hear the radiologist repeat half a dozen times "you have breast cancer Branwyn." I was unable to speak, and my husband fell to the ground and started to cry after hearing these words. So, what did I do? I hung up the phone and comforted him. I am a nurturer, cannot stand to see people hurting even if I am too. I sat there hugging him saying "I will fight Phil; I will fight." Fighting is exactly what I did. Through my entire journey I learned some incredible things about myself. If this diagnosis didn't happen, I never could have imagined what I would be capable of. I have come to realize that as absurd as this sounds - my cancer diagnosis truly saved me from having a nervous breakdown. That sounds crazy, right? But it is very true.

I felt a lump in my left breast on Nov. 29, 2021, one day before my 40th birthday. Happy birthday to me, right? This diagnosis happened not even three months after my yearly gynecological exam, which brought normal results for my pap and no lumps of any kind during the breast exam. So, why am I feeling a rather large lump now? How did something form that quickly? I'm not sure I will ever be able to put into words how without even being seen by any doctor or having any test I knew; I knew in my core the first time I felt that lump that it was cancer. A strange sense of stillness washed over me, and I realized right then I'd be fighting for my life, and if possible, I'd win.

Hearing the words "you have cancer" stopped me in my tracks. My head flooded with thoughts of leaving my children motherless and Phil a single dad. We haven't travelled to all the places on our list. The thoughts were nonstop. I took a few deep breaths, my thoughts shifted, I began to think of my job, a job that was destroying me. I had a highly successful but extremely stressful 100 percent commissions sales job that had me constantly working, tending to others (not my family), running myself ragged daily, not sleeping. I was working all hours of the night, stressing, constantly stuck in fight or flight mode, worrying, not eating as well as I should, not exercising, feeling trapped and hopeless in a very toxic work situation.

I found myself screaming at the kids since my fuse was short or crying alone in the shower, closet or in the car going to or leaving clients. Not only was I not present as a wife but also as mother to my three amazing children or even a friend. I was all consumed by work, unable to ever turn it off, always expected to be reachable. Always missing special moments or events, and ones I did attend, I was so distracted to enjoy them. I had let my priorities become so skewed.

The pressure I was under on the daily from others, accompanied by the pressure I put on myself with negative thoughts and feelings about situations and my body were slowly killing me. I couldn't see it then, but I sure do now.

I know that the daily stress or the constant high levels of cortisol I always had running through my body didn't cause my breast cancer, but I know it didn't help. It took me being diagnosed with Stage 3 Infiltrating Ductal/Ductal Carcinoma: Estrogen & Progesterone positive HERS2 negative breast cancer to stop me in my tracks.

For the first time in forever I took a good hard look at myself and was in disbelief at how close I really was to a nervous breakdown. Dec. 10, 2021 was the official date I was diagnosed with cancer, and from that day on nothing else mattered as much as fighting like hell for my life. I didn't care about clients' needs, my boss calling to scream at me for this or that (this happened pretty much daily), scheduled meetings, client renewals - I could have cared less about them.

I am not sure if the stars aligned for me, the universe was giving me another chance to live life differently or if a guardian angel was looking over me. From the minute I called my OB to be checked, everything went so smoothly. Things moved so quickly I was almost waiting for something to get messed up somehow. Well, nothing did - from getting appointments with ease to being scheduled for a procedure immediately, meeting my team of amazing doctors, having an angel as my nurse navigator, no insurance issues or delays.

I know the way things happened for me isn't the norm, many run into roadblocks and delays. I do not know why things happened the way they did for me; all I know is how grateful I felt for everything to have gone the way it did for a journey I never wanted to be on.

Together my husband and I went to every appointment so we both could hear, understand the diagnosis, procedures, tests I'd need, what was happening and when. If we had questions or didn't understand what we were talking about, I knew I could call and be helped. The comfort that I felt towards each doctor was immediate. There was a level of trust that I felt, so I gave up control to let my team do what they do best: kill cancer. My team had some of the most forward-thinking, brilliant, compassionate, smart, sensitive and intuitive doctors I had ever met. I put my trust in them wholeheartedly.

As I mentioned, the only decision I was 100 percent certain of right from the beginning was to go flat after the bilateral mastectomy. At the first meeting with my surgeon, she began to lay out options which started with a unilateral mastectomy and removing the affected breast, the left one or remove both — a bilateral mastectomy. I gave my answer quickly - take them both.

Leaving one would cause me daily anxiety wondering - even obsessing - over if cancer would claim the right breast too. The next conversation was about different options for reconstruction or not. She started with what is called an Aesthetically Flat Closure, which is the removal of both breasts with no reconstruction at all. Side note: something I've learned from the many women I've met through this journey is that their doctors did not even discuss this as an option, or if it was brought up, they would refuse to do it or even better make you meet with a psychologist first (how appalling) to make sure you are of sound mind to make a decision for your body.

She started to speak about implants. Politely, I let her know I was not going that route ever. She asked if I at least wanted to hear about them. My reply: "Nope. I'm good." Reconstruction with implants starts with expanders (metal cages) to stretch the skin after surgery to get it ready for implants. Then after months you have surgery for the actual implant. I did not want implants in my body. They could rupture, flip, my body could reject them or make me ill. Then another surgery is required after 10 or 15 years to have them replaced - no thank you! We then went back to discussing the Aesthetically Flat Closure and the different possibilities of how my scars could look. Dr. Hansen assured me that at the time of surgery she would do the best options for me to cause minimal scarring. I had faith in her decision and that she would do what was best for me.

I was never someone who had a large chest, so the thought of being flat didn't necessarily scare me as much as I thought it would. Don't get me wrong; the thought of having major surgery to remove body parts scared the hell out of me especially since this was my very first one. Go big or go home, right?! When I woke up from surgery groggy, I was somehow still able to ask: "Did it spread?" She said it did to seven lymph nodes. I turned my head, threw up and passed out. Other than that, the surgery went smoothly. Now my job was to rest and heal. My mom flew in to help me and to make sure I did as I was told.

Before cancer, I was never a priority. What I needed didn't matter; how I felt didn't matter. I just had to keep going, not stopping. Maybe I never stopped so I didn't have to think about the fragile mental state I was in. But now I did the opposite, I asked for help, slept when I needed, did not push myself or be strong to prove I could handle things. For once I did what I was told - rest. Doing as I was told really helped heal not only my body but also my very busy, stressed-out mind. I made myself a priority - it did not feel selfish at all, it felt amazing.

Physically healing from surgery wasn't as terrible as I thought it would be. I'm thankful for that. Even though I was certain of my decision to stay flat, seeing my body for the first time was hard. I stood in front of the mirror staring at this new body. The old Branwyn was gone; pre-cancer Branwyn was no more. I cried, sobbed knowing I would forever look different. I would have to learn my new body, learn to be proud of it.

This was the first step of healing - acceptance of my new body, the body I neglected physically and mentally for years and years. I cried knowing that I truly am fierce and a force to be reckoned with. As I stood there staring at my breastless reflection completely vulnerable seeing this new body of mine with clearer eyes than ever before, I was proud of myself for all my body had endured thus far. Through my tears I thanked my body for its strength.

Yes, I decided reconstruction wasn't right for me, but I learned that there are many options available to me should I want to "have breasts." They are called prosthesis, and there are many kinds of them. When we spoke about Aesthetically Flat Closure being the direction, my doctor got me in touch with an incredible boutique that specializes in post-surgical options for breast cancer patients.

I went to learn what was available to me, and it was enlightening. I learned so much — from different bra options to the different companies that specialize in bras, camisoles, bathing suits, even lingerie for women who decided to go flat. I was very intrigued by how much was available for me as a flattie (that is the term we use). Being flat I was thrilled to know there are still options for me to feel comfortable, confident, proud, and dare I say even sexy about this new body of mine?

I have four types of prosthetic breasts. I was gifted Knitted Knockers - they are made with extremely soft yarn then stuffed with wool. Some feel like bean bags that can go in bras or bathing suits. Others are made from silicone, have different shapes and sizes to mimic real breasts; they look and feel very natural.

Another option is to have custom breasts made. Yes, you read that right. 3D technology that creates custom prosthetics just for you are fascinating; they fit against your body like a puzzle piece. I opted to get all types I've mentioned. I did this for a few reasons – first, all types were covered by my insurance (sadly, some plans do not only not cover the custom ones they do not cover any) and second because I wanted to learn about them all so I could advocate for women who are thinking about AFC, to let them know this could absolutely be an option for them. Using all the different options, touching, feeling firsthand getting experience with them so I can better educate others, letting them know they can go flat or have "breasts" if they choose too. For me it's like makeup - some days I wear them and others I don't.

Breasts never defined me; I felt blessed I was able to breastfeed my three children, give them nourishment and experience that bonding. Other than that, I do not need breasts to make me feel like a woman or whole. I look at it more as I got rid of two of my body parts that were trying to kill me.

This entire journey saved my life; cancer saved my life. It feels very strange to say, but it's the truth. I didn't love myself, treat myself right both physically and mentally. I spoke negatively about my body in ways that I would never allow my daughter, sisters, friends or whomever speak about themselves. I didn't appreciate all the people that loved me. I did not know how to be present in my life or even how to not stress over things that I couldn't control. I continue to work on acceptance as well as how to live a life after cancer. For me that includes weekly traditional and EMDR therapy, medications for my mental health and sharing my story with others.

I wasn't taking care of myself properly, taking things for granted, never slowing down to be present and appreciating all that I have. Cancer did that for me. I've learned the importance of self-care. It is not selfish; it's necessary. I've learned that asking for help does not make you weak. A job that is toxic and causes an unhealthy amount of stress isn't worth it, not for any amount of money.

Yes, I am still Branwyn, dare I say a better version of the pre-cancer Branwyn. I give myself credit, have more confidence in myself, radiate positivity and feel so joyful. I'm choosing to see the good in people, in situations, not immediately going to worst case scenario over everything.

I am not always in a rush. I have slowed down big time, able to appreciate many more things, see the beauty in them and enjoy the new pace of my life that is now my new norm. I look at myself now as stronger than before. Yes, I have scars, but they remind me how strong I am and how far I've come.

On this journey there have been ups and downs, good days and really hard ones too. There were days I was certain I would not be able to make it through, but somehow, I did. What helped me tremendously was allowing myself to feel the feelings, good or bad. If I needed to cry, I did. If overwhelmed with anxiety and not wanting to attend an event, I didn't. I am more vocal when it comes to feelings. I make sure to tell everyone I love them more. If someone does something that warms my heart, I tell them. I allow myself to feel the good and the bad. I no longer push down or ignore them, pretend I am alright when I am not — another difference between pre- and post-breast cancer Branwyn.

Out loud every morning I say, "thank you, thank you for blessing me with another day." Blessed with the chance to fight for my life after being diagnosed with cancer, I think of all those who weren't given a chance to fight or are currently battling and those warriors who fought but lost their battles.

I know how lucky I am to have been given the chance to fight, given a second chance in life to move on from things that no longer served me and focus on the things that do. I take this opportunity of life seriously, want to help as many women and men as I can, make sure that everyone diagnosed with breast cancer never has to fight alone.

It's my mission to make sure women know they have choices, that reconstruction or implants aren't the only ones. If the surgeon does not speak to you about all options, advocate for yourself or if you don't feel comfortable, find a new surgeon. Everyone, both women and men, must do what is right for them and their bodies, remember you do have choices.

My hope for anyone on their journey is that they know they can thrive after their battle. They can be happy, confident, even gain a newfound respect for themselves, their bodies and all that they've endured. I want to help women know they aren't defined by their breasts, that they too can be fierce, fabulous and flat like me, or fierce and fabulous, whichever they choose.

# 7

# FINDING STRENGTH IN VULNERABILITY

## BY DIANNE JACKSON

"What do you pair with a diagnosis of breast cancer?" Not exactly the question I assume the poor sales guy at the Liquor Control Board of Ontario was expecting, but that is what I found coming out of my mouth without so much as a blink of my eye on Feb. 22, 2016.

Before we delve into my story, let me introduce myself. I am a mother of two wonderful adult children. I am divorced but count my ex-husband as one of my closest friends. I am the third girl in a family of four sisters. I have worked in the Canadian travel industry for over 35 years and live in Ontario, Canada. I believe travelling this wonderful world of ours teaches us compassion, tolerance and an appreciation for the rich tapestry of world cultures. But the most profound "journey" I have taken is my cancer journey.

I have quoted the word "journey" as I always truly disliked that term for what we go through as we undergo a diagnosis and treatment and try to normalize the rest of life. I disliked it so much — my family would cringe if someone would come for a visit and, in an attempt to offer words of compassion — ask how my journey has been. I work in the travel industry; if there is not a plane, train, ship ticket and copious amounts of food and wine, it is not a journey. I will, however, in this story, use the one word that seems to be universally accepted to describe the path of fighting cancer, but please know I am cringing as I do it.

My journey begins in the annals of my family history, a history scarred by the painful legacy of breast cancer. My grandmother (36), my aunt (39), and my mother (42) all succumbed to this relentless adversary, leaving me with a heavy heart at the age of 16. I could probably write an entire book on how losing a mother can shape a life (good, bad or indifferent), but I think I will focus this chapter on my specific breast cancer story and not on how cancer has shaped my life holistically.

Back in the days of my mother, aunt and grandmother, genetic testing for breast cancer (or any cancer, really) was virtually unheard of. Fast-forward to my generation, and via genetic testing advancements, women could learn if they carried the infamous BRCA1 or BRCA2.

When my older cousin on my maternal side hit 40, she decided to join the family breast cancer business and found herself fighting what her doctors told her would be a losing battle. Yes, you heard that right. Due to catching the tumor so late in the game, they were not giving her much hope. Now, I could probably write many details about my cousin's story, but I was asked to write about my story, so the critical takeaway from sharing about my cousin is she was positive for BRCA1. A final note on my cousin: I am sure she was diagnosed about 20 years ago, and she is still here proving those doctors wrong.

When I was around 26, my family doctor, recognizing our family's extensive history of cancer, recommended I participate in a study taking place at a well-known cancer hospital in Toronto studying genetics and high-risk breast cancer. When they offered me genetic testing, I agreed and figured I was in line for the next BRCA1 gene rollercoaster. I knew that the mutated gene that caused breast cancer also could cause ovarian cancer.

Breast cancer could be detected early, and I was part of this study, so, of course, they would find it early. Unfortunately, ovarian cancer usually did not get caught until too late, with little to no screening available. My focus, for whatever reason, was to get the genetic testing so that I knew if I was going to be at high risk for ovarian cancer. I was ready to have a complete hysterectomy if required-- for some reason, not even a thought crossed about mastectomies. To my surprise and delight, the test returned negative — I had won the genetic lottery. Now, please do not get too comfortable here — genetics and cancer, it turns out, can be a bit unpredictable. If the story ended here, I probably would not have been asked to participate in sharing my journey.

So, from the time I was 26 to the age of 47, I had been to the hospital for a check-up almost every six months where my assigned doctor would do a physical exam of my breast. In addition, I had annual mammograms, ultrasounds and MRIs as needed to check and double-check every little lump, bump and abnormality. I was and am so grateful for those doctors who were part of the study. Most were family doctors who gave up time with their regular practice to check people like me (ticking time bombs?). I felt there was no way a pea-sized lump would get past my defense army. Could it?

When you are part of a study, every single little thing they find, they check and double-check. So emotionally, you go through times of waiting for test results, so scared that you will have to have that conversation with your kids that my mother had with me and my sisters. I vividly remember being convinced something was wrong every time, well, except for that one time in early 2016, the one time that mattered the most.

On Jan 18, 2016, I went for my regular mammogram and saw the doctor (she will always be in my prayers). We chatted the usual chat — meaning, "No, I am not worried about anything unusual. I do not feel anything." I was 47 then, and my risk had dropped to 20 percent based on science. I was going to be released to the care of my family doctor by 50.

I remember smiling, yet there was a slight feeling in my gut of fear simultaneously — I was not sure I wanted out of this safety net of a study. As the doctor did her routine physical exam, she felt something in the left breast: "Nothing to worry about, Dianne, but as you know, we check everything." Heck, that is why I am here, right? She scheduled an ultrasound.

Before this particular ultrasound, I often would bring someone to accompany me to keep the butterflies calm in my belly. This time, I knew it was nothing — I went alone. We were only playing it safe, right? In hindsight, boy, was I wrong!

Technicians cannot say anything to you when they see something on the screen or give any results, but the writing is sometimes on the wall — they are technicians, not Oscar-winning actors. Once the first couple of images had been taken, the technician left the room to get someone else to look. They then took turns moving the wand around, taking a few more images --- for the record, an ultrasound on your boob is not as exciting as when you are pregnant or exciting at all, if I am honest.

A few minutes later, they left, and then they brought in the big guns --- the actual doctor (radiologist). I will never forget the three of them standing there and saying, "We are sure there is nothing to worry about, but we need to order a biopsy." The funniest thing about this was my response, and I believed it: "Oh, that is OK. I have had this many times before ... No worries; let's be safe." I sometimes wonder, when they left the room, if they looked at each other and said, "How sad and naïve that one is" or something similar.

My results from the biopsy came in, and the plan was that I was going to the doctors myself — I just felt, like so many times before, it was going to be nothing. Remember, I had been part of this study being checked for almost 20 years. I had, at this point, undergone two rounds of genetic testing with negative results (every few years there is more research done advancing what they can detect), physically checked pretty much every six months and, all previous "things" had been nothing. So, why would this one be any different just as I was almost at what felt like the finish line of cancer free? By the way, in my head that was 50.

One hour before leaving my downtown Toronto condo, walking

down my stairs, I suddenly buckled — it was as if someone yelled inside my head. I had cancer, and I did not need a doctor to tell me.

I called my best friend/sister to see if she could swing coming with me to the appointment. I heard somewhere that you should always have someone with you. Please note I always did bring someone with me — I recommend it (even if they do not go in with you to the appointment).

I also received some great advice early from a friend that I, too, will recommend: Keep a log of all the dates, tests, appointments etc. You are your own project manager (oh, maybe I should say travel agent due to my industry experience) in this journey.

Once at the hospital, when they called me in for my appointment, I said to my sister, "If I am right back, all good. If they say anything important, I will come and get you." I waited patiently until the doctor came in, sat down, and just like that, I had invasive lobular carcinoma (estrogen positive, HER negative).

I quickly told her to hold on. My sister was with me, and I wanted to get her. She told me to sit. She explained it to me first, then said, get your sister and I will explain again. I think she did that, so I heard it all twice; so that only my questions and concerns came out first.

I was so calm. I did not cry; I just listened. The doctor asked if I already knew. "Yes, can I go get my sister now so she can hear something different than I just heard?" I laughed. When I went to the waiting room, my sister smiled at me, thinking it was good news since I was longer than expected. All I did was shake my head no. I will never forget Linda's face at that moment. Our childhood fears had just come true. The doctor took her time and explained it all again.

Breast cancer, like many cancers, does not discriminate and is a versatile adversary — it can take many forms. When we hear breast cancer, we have all been conditioned to think of lumps. Lumps are the poster child of breast cancer, the rockstars of the tumor world. The peas in our breast that, if left unattended, grow to the size of a grapefruit.

Remember, we are talking about cancer, cells that have eluded the medical world for centuries. Invasive lobular carcinoma is one of those pesky forms of cancer that wants to play hide and seek. It does not grow in a ball; it forms a line of cells, tough to pick up on mammograms, ultrasounds and MRIs. The HER negative was good news as it suggests it is not too aggressive, and the estrogen-positive meant it grew in a rich estrogen environment.

My sister cried as the doctor explained it all. I sat and listened again. They were setting me up to see a surgeon the next day. At the end of the appointment, the doctor laughed and said, "Dianne, I think you need to take Linda home. Stop and get some wine — let it sink in. You have a rough few months ahead."

And so it began.

Due to the type of cancer, the doctor and surgeon wanted to verify the size utilizing an MRI. The ultrasound identified a growth of around 2 cm. This would be considered Stage 1, requiring a lumpectomy and probably some radiation. I had many friends and colleagues, including my mother-in-law, who had been through this, and I knew I would withstand this inconvenience. I would follow in the footsteps of my cousin — not the other incredible women in this now as I refer to it "family business."

My MRI proved to show just how very clever invasive lobular carcinoma is, as it had made its way from the outer edge of my left breast right across and over to the inner edge of the breast. In fact, when we got the pathology results after my bilateral mastectomies --- that little F-r (excuse my language) was 7 cm long!

On average, it takes this type of cancer about one year to grow a centimeter. Let's do the math: I had a 7 cm long tumor that would have taken about seven years to develop. OK, stay with me here.

Let's recap: every six months for the last 20 years, we were taking pictures and engaging in this game of hide and seek and heck, let's be honest, it probably thought it was going to win the entire game.

With this additional information, my treatment plan was far more aggressive than I had ever anticipated. I went from a lumpectomy and radiation to five rounds of chemotherapy, Twenty-five rounds of radiation, seven years (they wanted 10, but I made them give me the stats of survival without reoccurrence, and so we settled on seven since it was insignificant) of hormonal therapy.

So, in May 2016, my body was forever changed.

I pushed to have both breasts removed and later learned from my medical oncologist that my forever-surprising type of cancer is also one of the only breast cancers that may present itself in the other breast. Six weeks after the surgery, I started the chemo lounge, then moved to the radiation clinic, and just recently, I ended the hormonal therapy.

The battle against cancer is not just a physical one; it is a mental and emotional one as well. And that is where the power of resilience comes into play. It was my family's history, my mother's memory and the support of my loved ones that helped me muster the strength to face my cancer head-on.

The chemotherapy and radiation took a toll on my body and still does today but my spirit remained unbroken. The road was arduous, but I trudged forward with determination. My sister, friends and children, who stood by my side throughout the ordeal, were my pillars of strength.

Cancer stripped away some of the layers of my life and has forever changed me, but it does not define me. I found it left me vulnerable, but in vulnerability, I found a well of strength I never knew existed in me. I have now raised over $100,000 to support cancer research by participating in fundraising events.

I have offered my services as a "friend" to listen to people who need to talk to someone who may not have the same story (no one's cancer story is the same as another) but can relate. I have provided some interviews sharing my story in hopes of spreading the need to have women be educated to not always look for the peas or lumps — they may never find them.

It has now been seven years since my diagnosis, and even though this is my story, you must have already noticed that one person's journey touches so many people. There are people going through the battle with cancer, and there are all those people who have chapters as part of that story. The chapters on grandmothers, aunts, mothers and cousins. Stories of sisters, friends and children who watch you struggle both physically and emotionally. Stories of future diagnoses. Cancer is never just about the person hosting the cancer party — but it touches that person's community.

Note: I have now been tested for all 18 mutated genes that can cause any cancer; they all returned negative.

# 8

# 'YOUR SON HAS LEUKEMIA'

## BY JOSH TEHAN

Cancer. One of the most impactful words in human existence. No one is ever prepared to hear that someone they love has a life-threatening illness, especially a parent. Never in a million years did I think that my child would ever get cancer. Then the unimaginable happened.

My son, Ethan, was born in January 2006 and over the following four years, he lived a healthy and happy life. At the age of 4, he was your typical boy filled with energy and curiosity. He enjoyed going to preschool and playing with all his friends. However, in the early summer of 2010, we noticed a sudden change in his level of energy. At times, playing sessions were cut short as he appeared to be very lethargic.

While kids in his class were out at recess, he was taking a nap. It definitely wasn't normal for children his age. His lack of energy was also accompanied by a fever, and he began having sharp pains in his legs. All of this prompted us to take him to his pediatrician, who diagnosed him with having a common cold and growing pains.

These symptoms gradually worsened over the next couple of months, and our son continued to experience severe bone pain in his legs and pelvic region, a high fever and persistent fatigue. It wasn't until one evening, when he and I were wrestling around, did it boil over.

He completely stopped midway, laid on the couch in the fetal position and cried in pain that his "butt hurt." His temperature spiked quickly, and we decided it was time to take him to the emergency room.

Not long after the bloodwork was complete, the doctor entered the room and explained the results, which ultimately reflected abnormal white blood cell counts. From the look on his face and the tone in his voice, he knew something was very wrong. Without explaining further, he immediately had an ambulance take us to Inova Children's Hospital to run further tests.

This is the point where I believe everything began happening fast and life started to proceed in a completely different direction.

For three days from our arrival, he went through a long series of tests, which I can only describe as controlled chaos. With the testing schedules and level of worry, we hardly slept. Some family members were with us during this time as everyone was very anxious to find out what was wrong.

Finally, the head pediatric oncologist pulled us (mom, dad and grandmother) into a room to utter the gut-wrenching words: "Your son has leukemia." This is a moment in time that is forever engraved in our heads. Even to this day, when I close my eyes, I can still see the hospital room where the dreadful news was delivered: white walls with nothing on them, one desk, a sofa and two chairs. The essence of the room was a perfect depiction of the emptiness we felt when we heard those words.

I remember holding tightly onto his mom's hand and instantly feeling numb. The cries of my son's mother and grandmother were like no other. It was a level of pain that can only be exerted by any woman of motherhood. I felt for them, too.

For me, I went completely numb. The shock level was so high that I think it delayed the other emotions from occurring. However, as soon as the numbness subsided, that's when the denial, fear, anger and sadness rushed in. I was in complete disbelief and had so many questions. How could my son have cancer? Why does he have it? What is leukemia? Did we not catch this soon enough? Is it life-threatening?

Through all the noise in my head, I faintly heard the doctor instructing us to begin treatment immediately through a specific treatment program that was reliable and successful for his age and diagnosis. Then he requested we sign documents on the spot so they can get begin treatment. No time to think. No time to waste. We are now at the mercy of the doctors.

Now, how do you tell your child?

The most challenging moment that eventually snowballed into many challenging moments was that initial discussion with our son. After having to make several painful calls to family members, it was time to share the news with our son. How do you tell a 4-year-old he has cancer? As parents, we do everything in our power to protect our children. Now, we find ourselves by his hospital bedside, feeling a loss of control and having to deliver the worst news as best we can.

But before we could even speak a word, he asked, "When are we going home?" Holding back tears, we responded, "We are going to be here awhile because you're sick, and they want to make you better." Come to find out that "awhile" turned into a three-year battle. His chances of experiencing the joys of being a kid were now replaced with an arduous fight against life's worst enemy. I don't know another parent of a child who has cancer that wouldn't change places with their child in a heartbeat.

Soon thereafter, the doctor presented to us the treatment roadmap. Staring us in the face was a two-year program outlining phases of the treatment. Never in my life would I have imagined looking at a roadmap and thinking to myself that this is his new childhood journey. We see it on paper, however, neither of us was prepared for what was about to happen next.

The hard days were officially upon us as we embarked on the beginning of many phases of treatment. The first was a heavy line of chemotherapy and steroids. If it wasn't for the "So Your Child Has Cancer" (tongue in cheek) binder that was provided to us, we would have completely been left in the dark. We educated ourselves with the particulars of the chemotherapy drugs, all of which damages healthy cells as well as the leukemia cells. With that being said, the first 30 days of treatment were relentless. Honestly, they were downright brutal. Within the first few weeks, we witnessed the physical toll on our son and the many side effects produced by the chemo medicine. He consistently had nausea and vomiting, fatigue, loss of appetite and fluctuations in his blood counts.

Having to watch your child physically deteriorate was one of the most heartbreaking events no parent should ever have to experience. One of the most synonymous physical changes that happened during this time was the gradual loss of hair. So, to lessen the emotional pain, we decided it was best to shave his head. For me, it's cancer's form of branding. It has officially made its mark.

Unfortunately, this was just the beginning. The past month was an absolute blur and was full of "manys." Many sleepless nights, many tests, many emotions and many questions.

We found ourselves on information and emotional overload. This is when the support of family and friends plays an intricate role. Specifically, Ethan's grandparents. They were absolutely crucial to our mental, emotional, and physical well-being.

We took turns holding things together and holding each other up. Sometimes it was mom, me or one of our family members keeping it real to hold us together. Sometimes, it was Ethan. We were a team, and we had to be to handle everything that came down the road in our son's cancer journey. Because what came next was not on the roadmap.

During his cancer journey, we faced several challenges, and we soon learned that there is no better preparation than just taking it day by day. Each day was something different. Yes, we lived with fear and uncertainty all the time, but we had to continue to stay positive, educate ourselves and keep moving forward.

The everyday tasks were daunting enough. His full schedule of spinal taps, chemo regimen, bloodwork, just to name a few, kept us in a constant state of stress and worry. Not to mention the physical toll it had on our son. His legs were so weak from the side effects of the chemo that we had to carry him up and down stairs. Just walking for him was a difficult task.

Before I get into some of the non-roadmap challenges, I want to mention some of the outside noise. One of which was the stress of medical expenses and insurance issues. This was ongoing for years and requires a whole separate discussion, but I digress.

As far as work, we were fortunate to have jobs that were flexible with our schedule and made it easy. Some parents that I witnessed in the hospital weren't so fortunate. Imagine having to work long hours to cover the medical costs in exchange for time with your sick child? That's another hellish experience for a parent to endure.

Pivoting back to the non-roadmap challenges, our first involved a serious infection. Around the beginning of his treatment, the doctors surgically implanted a central catheter, known as a PICC line, in a vein above his heart so that medicine can be administered more efficiently through a port. Something we learned to do at home as part of his in-home care routine. An important part of this task is to ensure that the PICC line is kept clean to avoid infection. His immune system was consistently weak so we were doing everything in our power to steer clear of him getting sick. As part of the task of administering his medicine, we had to "flush" the IV line thoroughly with saline and de-access the port. This is not always foolproof, and he ended up getting an infection. It's very dangerous if it ends up in his blood stream.

After several attempts to inject antibiotics, it did not resolve the issue. The doctors decided to remove the infected line and insert a new one, hence adding another surgery to our son's resume. By the way, watching your child being put to sleep never got easier.

Along the course of his treatment, he ran into "smaller" challenges such as low blood platelets from the chemo, low oxygen levels in the blood and side effects from the steroids. However, none were more challenging than having to decide on whether to extend his treatment another year.

In the fall of 2011, things were starting to look up, and we were past the halfway point in his treatment program. The chemotherapy cycles were not as intense, and the healthy days started to outweigh the sick days. Ethan was home more, attending out-patient visits and following the roadmap. However, in December of that year, we discovered an error in the dosage amount of his steroid medicine that was prescribed. He had been taking less of the proper dosage associated with the treatment program.

Before this happened, we were always on top of the roadmap and hospital staff, making sure we were sticking to the script and getting our son the highest level of care possible. Minimizing any mistakes that could jeopardize his well-being. When your child is diagnosed with cancer, you have to be their advocate. One of our roles as a parent is to be your child's voice.

We never shied away from asking questions. We inquired with the clinicians as to what they were doing and why. Constantly finding out what can be expected from a particular procedure, what side effects there may be or what will happen after your child leaves the hospital. We ruffled some feathers at times, but sometimes we had to challenge doctors and nurses about decisions being made or medications being given.

We checked medications, monitored fluid levels in the IV bags, checked injections before they were given. We were the junkyard dogs always on guard. We checked everything, every time, all the time. So how did we miss this? Did we catch it in time? And most importantly, what happens now?

After the back and forth blame game between us and the hospital staff, it was discovered that there was a communication breakdown between the doctors and the pharmacy. But this was beside the point. Now we are left with the decision on whether to continue with the current roadmap or add another year to his treatment. Which meant that he was going to have to endure more chemo. This was by far the hardest decision we had to make. And at the end of the day, the one who is impacted most is our son. After deep conversations with family and doctors, we determined that it would be best to extend his treatment and hope that it achieves the same outcome we sought after.

When we suffered this setback, it was demoralizing. Sure, we reacted to the extreme disappointment that any parent would in this situation, with anger and hostility. But we knew we had to act quickly, re-group and set a new goal for his plan.

One thing that Ethan taught us through his entire cancer journey, even at his young age, was to smile through adversity. I recall one specific moment, when his mom and I were spending the night in the hospital to help monitor him. He had another grueling day of chemo treatment and needed all the help and support he could get from us. He was too weak to get out of bed in the middle of the night to use the bathroom, so we had to hold him up in his bed so he could urinate. As he stood there holding onto both of us to balance himself, he smiled so big and uttered, "I love you." It was at that moment we knew he was going to be someone special, and we were going to persevere.

As our son got older, we have watched him selflessly share his story with others to offer them hope, support and friendship. I've never witnessed Ethan complain or ask, "Why me?" Our son may not recall much. However, as a parent, it's a scar we have forever.

If there is one thing I can say about his cancer journey, it would be that there were just as many joyful moments as there were unhappy ones. Yes, I hated that the cancer seemed ever-present, even in the joy. But there were plenty of moments where love and laughter shined so bright that cancer couldn't dim it.

One humorous story that I remember to this day is when Ethan was home with his grandfather doing homework that consisted of using candy corn as part of the project. At the time, he was on a steroid regimen so you can imagine that he had quite an appetite. His grandfather looked down for one second and the next thing he knew, the candy was gone. Ethan had eaten his homework!

Although I have so much more, I share some of my son's story from a parent's perspective with the hopes that it resonates and exemplifies the very definition of healing, hope and resilience. As I look back on his successful battle against cancer, I learned a lot about cancer and its profound influence on everyone around it. During that journey, we learned the worst of cancer:

- Cancer is hard, brutal and relentless at times.
- Hospital stays are long. So are the effects of chemo.
- There are so many moments of childhood experiences lost.
- We experience fear and isolation.
- Tubes, wires and fatigue follow them wherever they go.
- We, as family members, quickly became "doctors" ourselves.
- Lastly, having to watch your loved one in pain.

However, it also revealed that through the physically and emotionally draining times:

- We laughed, we cried, and we discovered what quality time meant.
- We met some incredible heroes along the way: Patients, doctors and nurses.
- We learned a ton about leukemia and its impacts, both immediate and lasting.
- We shared stories with others and helped those in need.
- We became forever involved in the cancer community.
- We learned that together, we are not powerless. It takes a team of family, friends, hospital staff and more to fight.

How can I possibly communicate how my child's diagnosis and journey with leukemia changed my life? Without a doubt, it's difficult to convey the devastation we felt as a family in being unable to "protect" Ethan from the suffering he endured during treatment. This has allowed us to lean heavily on one another and trust the process.

I learned that we are not in total control of our lives as it consistently challenges us to persevere, stay positive through adversity and enjoy the little moments.

Looking back, I realize that you never know how strong you are until being strong is the only choice you have. So, if you ever find yourself in a similar situation as ours, or are in the middle of dealing with it, remember to enjoy the little moments in between the dark ones and continue to bring the fight to cancer.

# 9

# IT TAKES A VILLAGE

## BY KIM DUNPHY

Editor's Note: I received a message from a Kim Dunphy on Facebook a few months ago. It reads this: "A couple of hours ago there was a knock at my door and much to my surprise a package had been left on my doorstep! It was from Kathleen Chizak, who apparently, is a good friend of your parents. Knowing I am soon to be undergoing CAR T-cell treatment, she sent me a lovely shawl from a Ministry of Love and Connection in Hartford, Conn., and she included a copy of your book Perspectives on Cancer (Vol. 1). I sat down immediately, wrapped in my lovely soft shawl, knitted by praying hands and read the inspiring stories you included! As my team has advised me to keep a low profile to avoid contact with any viruses, I was looking for something to keep myself busy while I wait for my treatment to start next Wednesday, and I thought that you might be interested in my cancer story!" I immediately reached out to Kim to let her know I would be honored to include her story in Vol. 2 of "Perspectives On Cancer." Note: Kim's condition has improved since writing this chapter.

After 30 years of a somewhat tumultuous marriage, I had remarried a wonderful guy named Frank. After just a few short weeks of marriage, Frank needed a heart valve replacement. When he recovered, we started to travel.

For the next 14 years, we visited many countries, including Australia, New Zealand, Fiji, China, South Africa, Poland, the Czech Republic, Thailand, Croatia, Bosnia, Israel, Egypt, Palestine, Nepal and many more! We had a wonderful life together. What a peaceful existence!

We were both retired and moved to a lovely home in Summerfield, Fla., where each night we would take our tea outside and watch the sunset. Besides travel we would also visit our children and grandchildren in Baltimore, Md., and Walnut Creek, Calif.

As a first-grade teacher most of my adult life, I loved getting down on the floor and playing with the little guys! One weekend in California I took my grandson, Meyer, for a walk. On the way home I felt very tired, and at one point I fell down. He helped me up, and when we got back to the house, I remember wanting to take a nap. However, when I looked at the staircase to the bedroom, I felt like I was staring at a mountain.

I was just too exhausted to climb the stairs, and so I crashed on the sofa. This was very strange as only weeks before I had been climbing through the tunnels of Cappadocia in Turkey. My son and his wife were concerned and suggested I see my doctor when I got home.

When I arrived at my appointment, I explained my exhaustion to my doctor. I had used him for the last 10 years or so, and we had a great relationship. He ran all sorts of bloodwork, and his conclusion was that at 68 I could not expect to have the same energy level I had always had.

I went back with the same complaints a year later, and tests still showed I was perfectly healthy. At this point, the doctor was thinking that I was a hypochondriac. His assistant agreed to run some extra tests including a CT scan, but once again, I was a specimen of perfect health.

On a trip to Baltimore I noticed a severe pain in the scapula, which I decided was from hoisting my suitcase into the overhead bin on the plane. The pain got worse, so I finally decided to try a chiropractor.

After several treatments he suggested I get an MRI. Of course, the protocol is that you need to first have an X-Ray. Off I went with the order for the X-Ray, and the following day I picked up the written report that said, "unremarkable."

My doctor then ordered physical therapy. I went one day, and they had me using some sort of pulley. I have a high tolerance for pain, but it brought tears to my eyes, and I told the physical therapist I was done.

I went from that office directly to a walk-in clinic where I had experienced great care from their nurse practitioner. I explained to him my exhaustion and my pain level. He immediately called the facility where I had had the X-Ray and demanded they do an MRI. He is generally a jovial, positive person, and when they refused saying the X-Ray showed nothing, I heard him actually yelling into the phone that he was sending me over then and there, and they better do the test that evening.

It was 4:45 p.m., and they closed in 15 minutes. They begrudgingly put me through the MRI. I had told the technician that I was supposed to leave for Mongolia that Friday and was afraid to go with this severe pain as I would be riding horses and camels in the Gobi Desert with a backpack on my back. We laughed about that.

When the scan was completed, I could see her on the phone. The facility had closed, and we were the only two left in the building. She came back in and asked if I minded if she gave me contrast and did another scan. I knew she'd seen something.

Ordinarily, the technician tells you nothing and you have to wait for the radiologist to read the results. I did ask her if she felt it was safe to leave on my trip in two days' time. She suggested I go but see my doctor the minute I got home. That wasn't good enough for me, so I finally persuaded her to tell me more.

She took me into her room and showed me the original X-Ray and the MRI, both of which showed a distinct tumor and break in the bone. Somehow the radiologist had missed it!

The next day I went back to the walk-in clinic, and the nurse practitioner looked at the CT scan results on the computer and immediately took me into what I call "the inner sanctum."

He called the facility and demanded the original report from the X-Ray and the written report of the MRI to be faxed to him.

They said they needed more time, and he told them they had 15 minutes. The X-Ray report had an added line stating a recommendation for a follow-up MRI. What they didn't know was that I had already picked up the original report without the added suggestion.

I knew the results were not good.

The nurse practitioner told me I needed to see an oncologist immediately, and he called a friend of his, Dr. Maen Hussein, who agreed to see me at 7 a.m. the following day. By the following evening I was having a PET scan at 5 p.m., which I thought was odd.

Once again, the facility was empty except for a nurse and the technician. After the test was run, they sat me down and basically apologized for the mistake the radiologist had made. His photo was already gone from the "wall of radiologists." I believe they were really worried about a lawsuit. I told them no worries. I apparently had a fight on my hands, and I did not plan on adding a legal battle to the mix! I was then referred to Moffit Cancer Center in Tampa, Fla., and thus began my battle with multiple myeloma. NO GOBI DESERT!

At Moffit, I was seen by the multiple myeloma specialist who naturally ran all sorts of tests. It turned out that I am in the 1 percent of multiple myeloma patients who are non-secretors, and that is why the disease was never picked up. It would not show up in bloodwork or urine samples.

A bone marrow biopsy was the only predictor, and as it is pretty invasive, I guess my doctor did not see any reason to require that. I probably had this disease for the last two years. After receiving all the results, I was told I needed to start on radiation for the tumor and chemotherapy to reduce the number of cancer cells in my bone marrow to enable me to have a stem cell transplant.

There had never been any cancer in my family. I'd never smoked a day in my life, I was active physically and made sure we ate nutritious meals. The hardest thing at that point was having to call Zoe, my 7-year-old granddaughter and tell her I would not be flying up to Baltimore to attend "Grandparents Day" at her school, which I had done every year since she was in kindergarten. She began to cry.

I asked to speak to her mom and suggested my daughter try to gently explain that this wasn't a choice on my part but I would be busy with some medical procedures. They were living in the City of Baltimore at the time, and when I would visit, I would usually walk to the end of their block and cross the street to enter the Baltimore National Cemetery. Given Baltimore's critical position as a railroad and seaport hub, the Union Army had always maintained a strong presence in the city. This national cemetery was established in 1862, although many Union soldiers had been buried at this site earlier than that.

The gated grounds are lovely, quiet, and there are always several workmen around, so I felt comfortable taking her there. I read the sign at the entrance the first time we went and explained what a cemetery was and that we had to be respectful and not run around. Right away, Zoe picked out one particular grave of a World War I soldier, and every time we went, she would pick up any flowers that had blown off other graves and decorate the grave of James Henson. She did this on every visit and would "chat" with James.

That afternoon my daughter put my 4-year-old grandson, Jasper, in his stroller and walked the kids up to the cemetery. Having a degree in Public Health and working for an NGO in that field, Anne was not one to mince words.

She apparently sat both kids down and explained that "Nanny" had just been diagnosed with cancer, was needing treatment and that was why she would be missing Grandparents' Day. Zoe was very concerned.

Later that evening Anne heard her crying and went to comfort her, at which point Zoe asked if she could get out of bed and go make Nanny a card. Anne called me the next day and said Zoe had made me a drawing, but she was not sure if she was going to mail it to me. "Why not??" I inquired. Well, apparently Zoe had drawn an entire page of headstones with the different emblems of belief markings she had seen on her visits — Christian crosses, Judaism Stars of David, Muslim Crescent and Star, etc... I told Anne to look at each headstone carefully, and if my name wasn't on any of them, to send it to me. Thus began my somewhat humorous approach to my diagnosis!

Frank was by my side every step of the way, and the staff at Moffit began to call him my "bodyguard." During this phase, I was determined not to look or act sick. Each day I was scheduled for treatment I got dressed up, put on a little make-up and cool earrings. One nurse finally asked me if I was still working. I told her I was retired, but this was my job now and I planned to "dress for success!"

She gave me papers on a class they were having on looking your best. I loved it. I went to it with a couple of other gals, and we were given lots of free makeup and shown how to apply it. We also got to pick out free wigs and learned to tie scarves in the event we were to lose our hair. What fun!

I had to go through a series of tests at Moffit to assess my general health and make sure I was able to withstand the stem cell transplant. This even included riding a stationary bike and spending an hour with a psychiatrist. I don't remember what he asked, but he was laughing when I left.

I passed all my tests with flying colors and was scheduled for the transplant. I went home, and as I knew I was going to lose my hair, I matched all sorts of cool outfits with colorful scarves.

Frank and my sister, Cindy, were to be my caregivers, and in mid-February we all moved into an apartment minutes from Moffit Cancer Center. The procedure was pretty arduous. I had to take a shower every morning in special soap and be at the hospital by 7 a.m.

After a few days, I really didn't care about matching scarves and outfits. I was too busy vomiting. At one point, they let me go into a bathroom by myself, and I woke up in an MRI machine and had very little use of my right side.

They did not see signs of a stroke, but for months afterwards I had to see a physiatrist (which I never even heard of before!). If I went to use my left hand to do anything, Frank would tell me to try with my right, so I'd pick up and hold a glass with both hands.

The port they had tried to put in got three clots in it, so it had to be removed almost immediately and a PICC line (peripherally inserted central catheter) was put in instead. Because of the clots for weeks I had to give myself Lovenox shots. Try doing that with your left hand if you're a righty!

Frank said he'd do it for me, but his face looked a little greenish and his hands seemed shakier than mine. I figured out how to do it, bracing my right arm on the arm of a recliner. Eventually I got the use of my right side back. I won't go into the gory details of the stem cell transplant but suffice it to say, I was in Tampa for two months instead of the expected one, and the day I left the nurses gathered around to tell me they had not thought I was going to "make it!" I think they might have actually had a pool going! Fooled them!

After my sister went back to her life (PS I've always believed that being the caregiver is worse than being the patient), Frank refused to leave me alone. He would not go to breakfast with his friends, which is something he usually did once a month. He would not go to the workout center and he even stopped going to church.

He was so afraid I would fall. We had been told that it took 100 days after the transplant to feel well again. Frank kept track and was constantly saying, "You're at 55 days, only 45 left!" He decided that after 100 days he would book us a trip to England, Scotland and Wales. My son and grandson had visited from California that weekend, and we had a fine time. They went home on Sunday, Day 99. On Monday, Day 100, I finally persuaded Frank to call his friend Don and go have breakfast at McDonald's, one of his favorite places.

The two guys were both devout Catholics and had been used to doing this once a month and saying the Rosary together. I promised I would just stay in my recliner and not get up while they were gone. The next day, Day 101, Frank decided we would go look at a continuing care facility he had looked at months before. They had invited us for lunch and a tour of the facility.

We drove out and had a lovely day, although when I looked at all the walkers, I was sure this was NOT something I wanted just yet in my future.

On the way home, Frank asked if there were any TUMS in the car. I asked if he was OK, and he said he'd just eaten a little bit too much at lunch. When we arrived home, we were greeted by two adult Florida sandhill cranes and their two babies.

We'd been feeding these two cranes and their yearly two babies for about four years. Frank had taken over from me when I was advised not to get near wild animals after the transplant. It was a riot - Frank, a retired supervisory special agent of the FBI, had taught these critters to do their "mating dance" before getting fed four times a day.

Folks would stop by in their golf carts just to see Frank flapping his arms and jumping up and down. He'd wait till the cranes followed suit and then feed them by pouring out a line of seed. I would sit in the picture window in the dining room and watch his performances each day. If we were ever late, the birds would let us know by pecking on that window. They were pretty annoyed when we arrived home late for their dinner that evening. I went in and got Frank the mug of food, and when he held it up - for the first time ever, one of the babies walked right up to him and stuck his long beak right into the jar. Frank came in all excited wondering if I'd seen it happen.

That evening Frank tucked me into bed and fixed the blankets so they weren't resting on my feet that were very uncomfortable from the neuropathy I had developed from chemo. He kissed me good-night, told me he loved me and that he was going to watch the Mass on TV and then come to bed.

I was asleep when he came in. In the morning, for some reason, I woke up early and tiptoed out of our room. I fixed our pill boxes and then called a friend to see if she would take a walk with me.

I didn't like to go alone and figured Frank needed his sleep. When I got back to the house, the four cranes showed up. I went into the bedroom and said, "Frank, your babies want their breakfast." His hand was slightly raised, and there was a little smile on his face. I called to him again and went over to touch him. He must have passed away in the night.

Day 102 the love of my life, my caregiver and best friend, was gone.

Don later told me that when they'd gone to McDonald's they'd discussed death. Frank had told him that he wasn't afraid of death, he only hoped he'd die at home in his bed. Two days later he did. I blamed myself. I figured being a caretaker was just too much stress for him. At my next appointment, Dr. Hussein asked me where my bodyguard was. I burst into tears.

He hugged me and said I shouldn't blame myself. He said Frank would want me to live a good life, it was his time, but he was just waiting till I reached the 100 Day mark, and he felt I could take care of myself. He asked if I was still doing our evening tea routine, and I said it was too painful.

He made me promise that I would go out that night with my cup of tea and watch the sunset. I was able to do it that night and every night thereafter.

It took me three months to prepare for a celebration of Frank's life. I wanted to do everything myself. I worked really hard to become computer literate enough to make a DVD of his entire life and put it to music.

In September, over 150 people attended his celebration. The strange part of this day came later that evening. The day Frank died, there was a police social worker in the house. Ocala, Fla., provides this service for sudden deaths.

At one point he told me four big birds were at my dining room window. I knew Frank would want me to feed them, so I put the seed out. They ate and left.

In the morning and for days afterwards I put the seed out. They never came back. After years of feeding them, they never came back. Did they sense their friend was gone? The night of the celebration of life (remember, this was three months since the last visit of the crane family), my family was seated around the dining room table when they said my jaw dropped. There were the four cranes at the window. All of us trooped outside onto the driveway. The four cranes lined up in front of us, did their dance and slowly walked away. They have never come back. To that date, I've never considered myself a very "spiritual" person, but part of me believes Frank was sending us a message!

For years I had belonged to a group of couples who went to the local little theater for a play and a dinner about every few months. One of my friends called one evening and suggested I get back to this couples group as two of us were now widows. She came and got me for dinner and wanted to surprise everyone that I was rejoining them.

One of the husbands had recently been diagnosed with cancer and was in a foul mood, apparently taking it out on his wife and anyone around him. They sat me next to him. Gee, thanks! He started bemoaning how unfair this was that he got cancer, and he was generally ranting and raving. I finally said, "OK, STOP IT!" I told him he was wasting what energy he had being angry and feeling sorry for himself. Cancer is the luck, or the unluck, of the draw! Pull yourself together use your energy to fight the disease. I understand his attitude did change a bit after that evening.

People think I'm nuts making cancer jokes and laughing about this, but laughter helps me. I was always known as the "poet laureate" of my school where I taught. They were always funny odes. I've written a few cancer poems and even sent them to folks, like my Congressman Jamie Raskin when he was diagnosed. Attitude is SO important, after originally being told I had three to five years to live, I'm about to enter my ninth year of being a "myeloma warrior!"

In order to be accepted for CAR-T, you must have tried all other treatments. I've been in remission a couple of times, but this kind of cancer is like the "diabetes of cancer"... no cure , but it keeps coming back, and each time you can try a different treatment for it.

When COVID hit and only patients were allowed in hospitals, I felt I couldn't ask someone to drive me two hours to Tampa and then wait in a hot car for hours for me to finish my treatment.

I then decided it was time to sell my home and move near my family. My daughter and her family live only 15 minutes from Johns Hopkins. I now receive my treatments at the Kimmel Cancer Center at Johns Hopkins. When my cancer became active again after the last treatment, I became eligible for CAR-T therapy. Chimeric antigen receptor (CAR) T-cell therapy is a type of immunotherapy that uses a person's own immune cells (T-cells) to identify and attack cancer cells.

A few weeks ago my cells were extracted from my blood through a process called apheresis. The blood was passed through a machine that collected the cells in a bag. The remaining blood was returned to me through a catheter. I was watched very closely by a nurse trained to use the machine and care for patients throughout the collection. It took about four hours.

The cells were then shipped to the lab to be genetically modified and frozen. They are now waiting for me in some Johns Hopkin's freezer!

On Nov. 24, 2023, I began three days of chemotherapy to help prepare my body to receive the modified cells, and then I will have two days of rest before the CAR-T cell infusion.

I will be receiving pre-medications to prevent and control side effects. The cells will be thawed out prior to the infusion and after the infusion by my team. They will monitor my vital signs frequently.

For the next four weeks I will need dedicated caregivers at home round the clock. My daughter and my sister, as well as a neighbor and good friend who is an oncology nurse practitioner will be staying with me at home.

During this time, I will have daily visits to the outpatient CAR-T center at Hopkins to monitor for possible side effects. My CAR-T team is trained to manage any side effects. As my friend, Val says, "It takes a village!" I am so lucky to have my team and my "village."

# 10

# STRENGTH DOESN'T ALWAYS COME WITH AGE

## BY PAMELA FORMICA

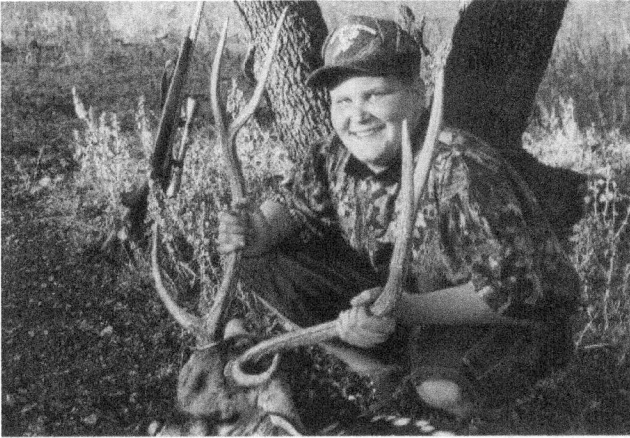

My son David was a typical 11-year-old boy; he led his football team in quarterback sacks, he took second place in district wrestling in his weight class and was a member of his school's undefeated basketball team.

I was the sports mom, that was until one game when my son got hit in the end zone and couldn't get up. More than that he got up crying. I had known for weeks that something just wasn't right. He had been to the doctor four times within eight weeks. Each time I was told to take him home and stop being an overprotective, overbearing mother.

But knowing something is wrong with your child and hearing that your child has leukemia is something that no parent can ever be prepared for.

On Oct. 14, 2002, my son was diagnosed with acute lymphoblastic leukemia. The doctors ensured us that if he had to have leukemia that this was the best type to have because it has a cure rate of 96 percent. David underwent 39 months of chemotherapy treatments that ended on Jan. 15, 2006.

He then started to live his life as he called "normal" when his leukemia relapsed on June 13, 2006, just five short months later.

He restarted chemotherapy treatments, and his sister Heather was found to be a perfect bone marrow match. David was scheduled to go for a bone marrow transplant over the Thanksgiving holiday of 2006. However, David had complications from his chemo - while his immune system was low, he contracted rhizopus in his lungs, which took his life five days later. David passed away on July 21, 2006, at the age of 15.

David was a compassionate soul. Even when he was diagnosed with leukemia, he told me that he was not mad at God because there are a lot of little children who have leukemia who will never be as fortunate as him to have 11 good years without it.

David never got to live life as a "normal" teenager, and he will never know what it is like to drive a car, go to the prom, graduate high school, get married or start a family.

The reasons that we need to find a cure for this horrible disease are countless. But numbers somehow always speak louder than words. David had a 96 percent rate of survival, only a 1 percent chance that he would relapse in his testicles and only a 25 percent chance that his sister and only sibling would be a perfect bone marrow match. Medical labs still cannot defeat rhizopus, which took his life.

I decided I needed to make David's death make sense, so I started raising money for the Leukemia & Lymphoma Society, not necessarily because my son was diagnosed with leukemia because I knew that the monies being raised would not benefit my son whether he survived his leukemia or not.

The reason that I knew I needed to help find a cure was clear to me on the day of my son's diagnosis when he looked up at his sister and me from his hospital bed and asked, "Am I going to die?" We answered him that day; we gave him hope by saying no - "No, David you are not going to die." That night I knew that I would someday envy the parent that could look at their child and answer that same question honestly and be able to sleep at night.

I gave my son hope in a small word, NO to his question.

No one knows if the next diagnosis is your son. We all believed at one time that cancer couldn't affect our families and never our children. This is not reality. There are not many people today that can say that cancer has not touched their lives or the lives of someone they know.

If you woke up tomorrow, what word would you need to find hope in?

My prayer is that someday that word is YES, yes we have a cure for cancer.

I work everyday to keep my promise to David to fundraise until we find a cure, I work every day so others' stories can end differently, better.

# 11

# CANCER IS A LIFELONG JOURNEY
## BY RUSS HEDGE

"*Perspective is everything when you are facing the challenges of life.*" - Joni Eareckson Tada

When you first hear you have cancer, it is a little shocking. My initial reaction was "no, not me. I am here to support others that have cancer."

God has blessed me with a good perspective on life and a positive mindset, which definitely helps, but even the most positive person doesn't want to hear those words.

I had been a supporter of others with cancer and specifically "Showing Up: Perspectives on Cancer" since the beginning. I was even blessed to be a guest on the livestream with Tim Sohn and Erica Neubert Campbell, talking about my dad's cancer and my role in his journey.

I lost my dad in July of 2017 to lung cancer. He was a lifelong smoker, so the cancer diagnosis was not a complete surprise, but it was hard to lose my dad. He was my hero and my role model.

He was originally diagnosed several years earlier and had major surgery. They took most of one of his lungs, and my family and I were there through a very long and rough recovery.

He got back on his feet, and even with some minor challenges, he lived a productive life for several more years. However, finally he was overtaken by cancer and dementia in the summer of 2017.

It was one thing supporting and caring for a loved one, but now, it was my turn.

Although I was dealing with a different kind of cancer, it was still life-threatening and a lot to deal with over the next year-and-a-half. In fact, like I said, I have learned that cancer is a lifelong journey - one I am still dealing with today.

My life as an inspiration specialist and entrepreneur was now being put to the test. I had to reshape my perspective based on my new circumstances.

I truly believe what Dani Johnson says: "You're not defined by your circumstances; you're defined by how you react to those circumstances."

It is true, as I always say: *"Life happens, and then you choose!"*

I had to make a choice. What was my next step after finding out life-altering information? Was I going to give in or move forward with my positive perspective?

It was definitely a defining moment.

I am a man of faith, and God has continued to keep me strong in all circumstances in my life, so why not now?

But it's not always that easy. How we react makes a big difference.

*"Life is 10% what happens to you and 90% how you react to it."* - Charles R. Swindoll.

So here is my story:

It was July of 2022, and I discovered a hard spot on the bottom of my foot. I asked my beautiful wife to take a look. She said, "It looks like a wart." Two months later I was diagnosed with cancer - stage 2A invasive melanoma.

The "C" word was alarming, but the way the dermatologist described it, it sounded fairly routine. I thought, "No big deal. They will cut out the cancer, and I'll be all good."

Because of my God-given perspective on life, I usually just roll with the punches. "It's all good" is my motto.

Like I said earlier, perspective is everything when you are facing life-threatening circumstances.

It is so much easier to have a positive perspective when life is good. It's when the challenges come that the rubber meets the road. It's how you bounce back after you fall down that matters.

*"It's not how far you fall but how high you bounce that counts."* - Zig Ziglar

I was referred to Oregon Health Sciences University (OHSU) to see an oncologist surgeon and a plastic surgeon. By the time my appointment arrived, about a month later, they found an additional spot of melanoma on my foot. I was told they would have to remove about half of my instep on my right foot, slide the other half over to cover the weight bearing portion and borrow skin from another area on my body to finish rebuilding my instep. It would be about a four- to five-hour surgery.

They would also remove a lymph node in my right groin area for testing, just to make sure the cancer hadn't spread. They felt very confident we had caught the cancer early, so the prognosis was good.

I had surgery on Nov. 11, 2022.

The surgery went well, and they sent me home the next day to begin the slow recovery process. We were all feeling optimistic.

I thought we had it all taken care of, and the pathology report would just confirm that. But, on Thursday, Nov. 17, I received some unwelcome news.

The day started off great at my post-op appointment at OHSU. I was told the cancer removal and the plastic surgery they did to repair my foot was looking good, that I was healing as expected.

After the good news, my beautiful wife, daughter and I drove home. I was tired but feeling great about the doctor's observations.

Then we got home, and I opened my email. I saw an OHSU MyChart message with the test results from pathology. I was expecting more good news.

The first part was great. The bottom of my foot where they cut out the cancer looked good. The outer tissue was cancer free. Very good news.

The next part was not so good.

In the lymph node they removed in my groin area they found a malignant tumor. My oncologist surgeon called a short time later. He informed me that meant the cancer went from Stage 2A to Stage 3C, very serious, and further treatment or surgery was needed. They were also doing additional tests and scans to make sure it had not gone any further in my body.

The news really shook me and my family. In fact, my son and daughter-in-law called from California to find out the results, and as I began to tell them, I looked up at my wife and daughter — both with tears running down their faces, and I lost it. I couldn't talk.

It was a life-changing moment.

I always look for the positive, and this was difficult, but God was going to use this experience to grow and guide me. He was going to help me to encourage thousands of people.

It was a pivotal moment, and one that took most of the night to recover from. But tomorrow was coming.

My dad, my hero, used to always say, "Tomorrow's a new day!" After a good night's sleep, the morning brings a fresh perspective.

I truly believe we have to experience the emotions of each situation, but as the saying goes, "time heals all wounds," and I knew I was going to grow through this experience and come out better on the other side.

I love the quote by Justin Winski: "Don't let your circumstances define you. You define your circumstances."

It is only God and each of us that define who we are and what we are planning to do with our circumstances. We have to be intentional in our life.

After the initial shock of the diagnosis, I felt God saying to me, "It is going to be OK. I've got this!" I knew God was not done with me yet. I had a peace about the cancer but knew I had more to do.

I truly live to Inspire and encourage others, and this cancer in my life would define all I said and did from this point on.

I believe life happens, and then you choose.

My why or purpose came alive. I believe I am here to inspire and encourage others to live a purpose-driven life of significance. To help people make a life changing impact and a difference now.

*"A life is not important except in the impact it has on other lives."* - Jackie Robinson

What is your impact on the lives of others?

What are you intentionally doing every day to make a difference and be a blessing to your fellow man?

*"In every day, there are 1,440 minutes. That means we have 1,440 daily opportunities to make a positive impact."* - Les Brown

That is amazing and a lot of opportunities most of us pass up daily. So you and I get to choose our path - the life we want to live.

In 2020, at the height of COVID, I wrote and released my first book, "Befuddled? Live the Life You Choose!" It was a book about living with purpose and a positive mindset, in spite of life's circumstances. I talked about perspective and how you look at life, especially through life's challenging circumstances.

I have had some big moments happen over my lifetime. I wrote about my near fatal car accident in July of 1983 when I was only 19. I've lost both my parents - my dad to lung cancer and my mama to Alzheimer's. All of this happened in the month of July, coincidentally the same month I found what we thought was a wart on the bottom of my foot.

Even though I lived through challenges, this was different. This really shook me to the core. A life-threatening, unbelievable disease was actually happening to me.

I first wrote about this journey in my last book "Rattled Awake," Volume One. That was an amazing opportunity, like this one for "Perspectives on Cancer," to collaborate with other authors and put together a book that will positively impact others.

My job as a marketing coach, keynote speaker, livestreamer and livestream producer, gives me many opportunities to speak to people. Whether it is online, in-person events, or through my writing, I am blessed to have the opportunity to speak into others' lives.

I want to be real in my communication as I feel authenticity is so important. My friend Nancy Debra Barrows would say, it was time to start #RadiatingReal.

I am blessed to be friends with Tim Sohn, the creator of the Showing Up: Perspectives on Cancer movement. I was able to recently attend a live conference in Scranton, Pa. What an amazing opportunity to be with cancer warriors, caregivers and supporters of the cause.

Any chance I have to impact others in a positive way, I'm all in. I continue to feel God using me to share my journey while displaying my positive attitude and perspective.

I try to always be honest and vulnerable and share how I am moving forward, even through ongoing challenges.

It is not easy at times, but it is an intentional choice I make each day.

The truth is, the challenges kept coming. After the first round of Immunotherapy, they found more cancer in the lymph nodes in my right groin. I had to choose to change drugs in my treatment, or surgery. After speaking with my oncologists and a weekend of prayer, I chose treatment.

My body didn't react well to the second treatment. I got extremely sick and contracted Type 1 Diabetes as my pancreas started to shut down.

I had to have another surgery to remove more cancer. It was an invasive surgery, and they removed 11 lymph nodes in my upper right groin area as well as moving a muscle to protect that area.

It was once again a long recovery, but with a great result.

About a week-and-a-half after the surgery, the pathology results came back, and they found cancer only in one of the inflamed lymph nodes, and it was contained. They had removed all the cancer.

They had planned to do radiation after the surgery, but the OHSU Tumor Board met, reviewed my situation and decided no more treatment was needed because I was cancer- free.

My story is ongoing, and I intend to keep encouraging and inspiring others through my actions. I am believing in God's complete healing, but at this point I am having to adjust my rhythm of life to deal with the diabetes.

I am also dealing with additional things the trauma of cancer caused in my body. I have internal digestive issues, and after many procedures and tests, they believe it is from colitis. For a while I was taking enzymes. They thought my pancreas was not providing for my digestion. I also have had vertigo and hearing and vision problems.

Cancer is a lot for your body to take, but whether I deal with this temporarily or for a lifetime, I will continue to stay positive and keep a good perspective, knowing God has blessed me far beyond my problems and challenges.

As the amazing singer Nightbirde said: *"I am so much more than my problems."*

Our story never ends, and the perspective we embrace will make a significant difference.

With a little imagination and commitment, we can do amazing things, in spite of our challenges.

*"The only limit to your impact is your imagination and commitment."* - Tony Robbins

Is today the day you decide to live your true, authentic purpose for life?

Whether it is cancer or some other life challenge that is getting in your way, are you going to let it stop you, or are you going to fight through and share a positive attitude and perspective?

You were blessed with the opportunity to do just that.

I believe life is truly amazing.

This messy life is worth the fight! Hold onto hope, and remain strong! There are awesome days ahead!

You can learn more and connect with me at russhedge.com.

## 12

# GET READY TO LEAD A LIFE BY DESIGN, NOT DEFAULT

## BY ZORAIDA MORALES

I never thought healing myself mentally, physically and spiritually after a cancer diagnosis would lead me to become a nutrition and cancer coach to empower and support cancer survivors and caregivers, but it did.

Why do I feel pulled to help 1.8+ million people diagnosed with cancer last year?

My why is simple...

I was diagnosed with chronic myeloid leukemia (CML) in 2008, am celebrating 28 months in remission and believe my life's legacy is to heal my cancer community when they need help the most.

Prior to receiving the cancer diagnosis, I lived to work and never considered working to live. I was born into generational poverty, so this convoluted way of living was normalized for me by my family, community, and environment.

To overcome these challenges, I went to college, worked long hours and rarely considered my heart and feelings when making life decisions. I was living a life fueled by the mind and ego.

Looking back, I thought I was living the American Dream of living in the suburbs, owning a home and being the proud mother of two young boys while working as a manager at a New York global financial services firm. What else could I possibly want or need?

While recovering from foot reconstruction surgery in 2008, I scheduled an annual physical like I did each year, expecting ordinary results.

But this time was different.

My primary physician noticed high white blood cell counts that were doubling and tripling each day.

Fear was setting in. My intuition told me this news was not good. But still, I was not going to react without proof. So, I went about life as though this was an inconvenience.

In my heart, I knew that life as I knew it was gone.

At the insistence of my primary care physician to get a proper diagnosis after days of multiple blood tests, I met with a local hematologist on Nov. 14, 2008. Did you know you cannot meet with an oncologist until you have a cancer diagnosis and you cannot get a diagnosis until you meet with an oncologist? It's the chicken vs. egg dilemma.

At this local doctor's office, I was informed I had CML and was immediately scheduled to have my first bone marrow aspiration and biopsy, which involved removing a sample of bone marrow and testing it for signs of disease.

You.

Have.

Cancer.

I felt a heavy weight when I heard those words. It landed like a seismic shock to my body. It was a challenging moment, filled with a whirlwind of emotions. It was like being caught in a storm where fear, uncertainty and disbelief collided. In that instant, my world shifted and a flood of concerns rushed in.

"What?!"

"I cannot have cancer. I have three- and six-year-old boys to raise!" I cried.

It worried me as I raised my voice.

I called my husband while I drove home, and we both sobbed as the rain pelted my car that Friday afternoon.

I felt assaulted and betrayed.

That evening after putting the boys to sleep, we held each other as we cried ourselves to sleep.

The bone marrow exam was performed with no anesthesia and no medication and lasted around 30 minutes. While I meditated through the exam, I remembered my husband gasping when looking at the length of the needles.

During the first six months after the diagnosis, I continued my college studies while getting into remission. I tried to live normally, but fear and worry took over my mind. I was grieving for my old life and was not mentally or emotionally ready to accept the diagnosis. I wanted my old life back.

You don't know what you don't know.

Our emotions were high with fear and anxiety mainly because the medical care industry does not have a blueprint to heal cancer survivors holistically, just medically. It's important to receive a diagnosis and medical treatment. Conversely, it's imperative to heal the whole person: mentally, physically and spiritually.

Fifteen years later, I see that as survivors holistically heal, we are showing the medical care industry that proper healing includes the mind, body and spirit.

I experienced five phases of grief: denial, anger, bargaining, depression and acceptance. While going through the motions of living with cancer, my past trauma and limiting beliefs made daily appearances while my mind was on overdrive. My heart was broken.

*"I'm not afraid of storms, for I'm learning to sail my ship."* - Louisa May Alcott

The breakdown prompted me to stop my college studies to focus on my mental health. It was time to wrap myself around the diagnosis because I was still in denial. I did not make the mindset shift needed to live differently with cancer. The hardest prison to escape is in our mind. My childhood trauma and limiting beliefs were not allowing me to move forward with the diagnosis.

The people around me, my husband, parent and siblings did not like the internal changes I was making because I was putting time and energy into myself.

My diagnosis triggered their own traumas. They did not have the emotional tools to give me what I needed, like help with the boys because they did not have that support given to them. I hosted fewer holiday events, stopped coordinating family travel, stopped giving my power away and said no often to prioritize myself.

I had to stop being me.

After the divorce and while packing up our New Jersey home during COVID 19, my boys haphazardly performed their chores, talked back and were resistant and ornery. They fraternized at colleges and played basketball with friends while I sold furniture to prepare for the sale of our home.

When we arrived in New York City, the difficulties continued. The boys did not unpack, throw out empty boxes or clean the kitchen after meals. To top it off, they were quick to set up the Xbox.

That was the last straw. I was so angry. I would no longer accept their insolent behavior. I told them they needed to leave immediately, that I was not going to tolerate their sh*t anymore. That was the most wretched day of my life.

All I could do was cry and scream at the guilt and shame I felt for removing them from our apartment. I cried, alone, surrounded by unpacked boxes.

I understand that the boys did not want to leave their childhood home and that the divorce was not their fault, but this was my first step toward protecting and self-trusting to begin the healing process, through a desire to be a better me.

I was not prepared for the painful feelings I felt after hearing my mother's unfiltered opinion to stand by my marriage, which then brought up memories of my childhood abandonment. She knew first-hand of the dysfunction in my 24-year marriage, yet she tried to convince me to continue in the status quo. How would staying in a toxic situation be good for me or the boys? And then I remembered that her emotionally absent father gave her similar advice when she initiated the divorce from my father in the late 1960s. It made sense.

"Are you listening to yourself?! You want me to stay with a man who does not value me and puts me in danger? This is your unresolved trauma talking! Don't project your sh*t on me!" With these words, I hit a nerve, and she hung up the phone. I cried and screamed, "How is this happening?" That's when I concluded that she did not always consider my feelings and did not always protect me during my younger years. I also had to take responsibility for the demise of my marriage as I came into it with my own trauma and with that epiphany, I joined a 10-month trauma program to break the generational karmic energies plaguing me.

Divorce affects all family members, and everyone in my family had an opinion. How dare I think I am enough to set boundaries to put my emotional and physiological needs first? This conversation reminded me that I was unhappy with our relationship for a long time. I had to step away because I could not grow if I continued to experience her negative behavior. The effects were holding me back, and I saw no reason to continue torturing myself. I separated from her to be in alignment with myself. I had to remove myself from her way of being to find the words to set boundaries while not letting her words hurt my heart.

Your own family will talk behind your back when you're in the process of breaking all their generational curses. This isn't for the weak.

As I find the words to be a responsive — not reactive — communicator, I continue to do the internal trauma work.

Setting myself up for success means I love myself, then love myself some more. I no longer look for others to make me happy because that gives others the power to make me sad. Being my own best friend and cheerleader is how I choose to live. I am parenting myself in the loving way I parent my children. That means I am self-loving, self-trusting and self-accepting and do not reflect negative emotions toward myself, and when I do, I quickly reframe the words. I AM WORTHY! I AM NOT MY PAST!

Mirror work is my powerful strategy for change. I'm lovingly redirecting my self-criticism positively to help me make better choices and resist discouragement, even when I have setbacks. I refresh my efforts and strengthen my willpower by understanding the circumstances in which my efforts sometimes let me down. This is the best gift I have given myself.

After forgiving others and myself, I wrote a poem on May 26, 2021, during the Full Moon Total Lunar Eclipse:

*I accept myself and what I participated in*

*I said what I said, I did what I did, and I understand that at the time that felt right to me, and at that level of consciousness I did not know better*

*Now I understand more of what my truth is and how I show up*

*I see it differently*

*I am a different ME*

*I am aware now and am bigger in my consciousness and in my heart*

*I will no longer hold myself hostage for my mistakes*

*I am healing across generational ancestors*

*I am not my past!*

*I am enough!*

*I will love myself, I love my life!*

*And so it is with Sirius Joy!*

*"The only way to make sense out of change is to plunge into it, move with it, and join the dance"* - Alan Watts

I made the mindset shift to have my heart lead and the mind and ego follow and support. In the past, I was solely working with the mind and ego; I was living in default. I was unhappy in my soul and did not know what I needed. I realized that overcoming feelings and emotions would lead to a revolution. Because, when the heart does not lead and the mind and ego rule, there will be trouble.

My ego was in cahoots with the mind and consistently ignored my heart's wishes. My mind would tell my heart to toughen up and stop acting like a baby, just push harder. The same words my mother used to motivate me as a child. My mind and ego ignored my heart wanting love from family and friends, giving my body rest when necessary and making excuses when family did not show up like I wanted and needed them to do.

Now, I have a better understanding of what my heart feels, needs and wants. As I understand the mistakes I made when not leading with my heart, I can see I was doing it all wrong. My mind and ego were putting my heart in difficult situations, rarely consulting my heart, being co-dependent on others and people-pleasing while giving my power away because of money triggers, limiting beliefs and trauma.

Now, my heart rules, and my mind and ego follow and support. It is where what I am feeling is trying to maintain emotional integrity, as it works to bring my mind and ego into integrity. Feelings are facing off with my other feelings. I know now that I must be gentle with myself and continue to self-love, self-trust and self-accept. I am attempting something great!

How did I want to live?

What was I hungry for?

What did I need but did not have?

And how do I get it?

I asked myself these questions. Because all I wanted was to live in peace, love and joy. But what did that look and feel like?

The answers came when I was asked to speak with the mother of a 27-year-old who was diagnosed with breast cancer. The mother wanted to learn how I moved through cancer and the important steps of living with cancer.

It broke my heart when she talked about the lack of mental health information she received from the medical team. She and her daughter were lonely and anxious and unfortunately did not have family and friends to support them emotionally. Sadly, it's common that many family and/or friends feel overburdened with the additional obligations when they are asked to support, as most lack the skillset to help.

I gave mother the space to break down, ask questions and presented her with my list of 7 Things To Do Following a Cancer Diagnosis.

Mother profusely thanked me, and at that moment my heart opened to accept her gift of gratitude. My heart lit up, my fingers tingled, and at that moment I knew I received the message from God

Universe that I was here to learn the path so I can teach others to increase their resilience, eat healthy and minimize anxiety while soothing the mind and spirit to see hope in the possible.

*"Into a daybreak that's wondrously clear, I rise."* - Maya Angelou

This was not supposed to happen.

Or was it?

I came home from a European study trip with a cast and crutches.

My foot was not supposed to give way when stepping on the edge of a ramp, spraining my ankle, causing my kneecaps to hit the concrete and tearing both menisci.

Once home, I found myself barricaded in my apartment, taking pain medication while revamping my calendar and wondering how I got here.

I needed to ask for help, to slow down.

You see, I was a doer and was not always good at asking for help.

Intellectually, I know that no one succeeds alone and collaboration is key, but I had a hard time asking for help, even though I was quick to help others. Growing up in a Puerto Rican household meant I was more comfortable putting others' needs first and mine last. I was not taught self-love. If I was going to learn the lesson and successfully shift from a financial professional to a cancer coach, now was the time.

A coach requires authenticity, feeling and empathy to earn the client's trust and rapport, and I was not comfortable with those emotions. Growing up, the people I asked for help were emotionally incapable of healthy modeling. They couldn't give what they didn't experience. I was discouraged to ask for help because that meant family secrets would be exposed and that brought guilt and shame to our family. Nipsey Hussle said, "If you look at the people in your circle and you don't get inspired, you don't have a circle, you have a cage." I recognized I was asking the wrong people for help; I did not have the right people in my circle.

Ahh, now I understand where many of my limiting beliefs were established.

Our secrets included emotional and physical abandonment,

poverty, lack of love, lack of safety and shelter, all low-level needs essential to reach self-actualization.

"Yes, you can call the ambulance" and "Yes, please follow the ambulance and stay with me," were the words I used when surrounded by these caring people. Though I was 4,000 miles away from home and did not speak Russian, Swedish, or Finnish, I felt supported and taken care of. I was not afraid. I said yes, and God Universe put these wonderful people in front of me to change my former beliefs. I learned that when you ask, people want to help. I AM Worthy.

My heart was not scared; my mind and ego did not conjure up negative scenarios but instead soothed my heart to come into alignment. I stayed emotionally and mentally balanced. It felt good to be in integrity; my fingers tingled. I was on the right path.

That was my biggest lesson this past summer.

Each time I expose limiting beliefs, I reward myself with the grace to take things slow, to take time to reflect and to devote more time to myself, so I can hear the intuitive messages.

As I ask for help, I realize I have come through to the other side, and with this new perspective see things differently.

Fighting cancer requires a mindset shift. This is where a coach is needed for the survivor to find the energy and space to move through surgeries, treatments, anxiety, fear and limiting beliefs.

Right now what I am passionate about is helping survivors using the Three Pillars of Nutrition in my cancer coaching business.

In my capacity as a coach, I help clients:

1. Establish their solutions and strategies
2. Support and believe in them, even when they may not
3. Help set and clarify the focus of the client's goals
4. By holding clients accountable for what they say they are going to do.
5. While meeting them where they are because they are all at different levels of consciousness

I provide the resources to navigate the unexpected road of cancer to move from the life they were born to, to live the life they were born to live.

I am right there with them managing my health.

My mission is to educate and empower cancer survivors and caregivers by walking alongside them using holistic tools to get ready to lead a life by design, not default.

# 13

# LOVE NEVER RETURNS VOID: THE GIFT OF SERVICE

## BY ARIEL "SAYEN GATES" & ELIZABETH LEYSATH

I had never truly contemplated the significance of my role as a servant to the people, but being in service to my family demanded a unique form of strength, one that I never realized I possessed until it was put to the test.

From a young age, it was instilled in me that God bestows various gifts upon His people, each with his or her own strength. Mine, I was taught, is the gift of service.

Whether my actions were directed toward others or my own family, they were consistently driven genuinely from the heart. My mother and Aunt Debra, in their wisdom, shared with me that gifts like mine are indeed a blessing, yet they come with a downside — not everyone will appreciate the depth of such a gift, and some may even take advantage of it. It was very important to grasp the distinction early on to prevent future harm; others shouldn't bear the consequences of your past actions.

From the late winter 2019 to early spring of 2020, I was working as a medical assistant/phlebotomist at Lexington Medical Hospital in Columbia, S.C., for the past almost three years. It felt like I had been there longer than that because of how much I loved the job and what I did, but I wanted to do more.

I signed up for school in August of 2019 to pursue a bachelor's degree in human services, I thought it would be something new and different to learn because I loved working with children and young adults since my service in the youth ministry at church. Plus, at my core, family is everything to me, so why not expand my territory?

My life has always been hectic and busy so sometimes it was hard for me to see family and friends due to my ambitious nature, but whenever holidays, birthdays or special occasions or random meet-ups came around, I'd always be there for the occasion.

While pursuing my career, I was also searching for a place of my own to call home. Having shared living quarters with my friend Malcolm for the past two years, I yearned for the independence and stability that a personal space could offer me. I looked at my chances as favorable, given my lengthy employment with the hospital. I thought it was safe to say that getting an apartment would be a no brainer. However, it proved to be more of a challenge than I thought, especially considering a new policy implemented by certain apartment companies in January 2019.

This policy stipulated that prospective tenants were required to demonstrate an income ranging from two to three times the monthly rent to qualify for approval. What initially seemed like a straightforward process transformed into an unforeseen challenge. Those conditions made it abundantly clear that the available choices were either rundown, unsafe or located in areas where even law enforcement hesitated to go.

After several weeks of relentless searching, I reached a decision to approach my mom and aunt. Temporarily I would stay with them until I secured a place where my biweekly paycheck of $639 would stretch further and provide a sense of financial stability. Thankfully, they agreed, under the condition that I cover a few household expenses.

In March, I made the move and settled into my old room near the front of the house. Nothing looked like it had changed much from when I was a teenager — from the hollow white walls to tiny closet where most of my mom's and aunt's clothes hang now. You could still see the tag from the dry cleaners on the clothes wrapped in thin plastic.

The blue industrial carpet looked like it hadn't been vacuumed in a while, which meant my allergies were going to have a field day. The tiny room gave me dread because of the memories in these walls, but I kept telling myself this is only temporary and soon we'll just be visitors again instead of occupants. Malcolm continued to check in on me periodically; he understood that being with my family was precisely where I needed to be.

In some way it felt like divine positioning, a preparation for the challenges that lay ahead, with my loved ones providing a foundation for outside struggles. God foresaw something even I didn't know — how much I'd be needed.

Now before we go any further, I want you to get to know a little bit about my family, especially who I'm writing about.

Debra Jean Leysath-Baker or "Deb" as we liked to call her was my aunt but more of a second mother and accountability partner in my life. Her essence and approach to me when I was having a good or even difficult time was the same as my father: non-judgmental, caring, and she never forgot to sprinkle the love on top.

I saw how she was able to help my mom smile more when I wasn't there, which was great because I worried about her. My mother Elizabeth is a private person, not afraid to tell you how she feels but always kept her feelings reserved. She loved me unconditionally like any mother would, but sometimes I worried whether she was happy.

I always tried to make her proud of my accomplishments whether in school or outside of it. Someone once told me that "to honor your parents is to show them that the teachings they taught you still live within in the vessel from which growth was sprouted."

Both my aunt Deb and mother feed our family spiritually, giving and providing wisdom that we all carry with us even to this day, and the fact that I have the honor to talk about her makes this even more special.

*Deep Breath* Let's begin...

In the cool month of March 2020, my mother noticed Deb

couching more than usual, and like she did with all of us as kids when we got sick, she'd give us medicine, rubbed VapoRub on our chests and under the nose to get the cold out. If it was really bad, she brought in the "big guns" like green rubbing alcohol, which to me kicks it out faster.

As a couple of days went by, we both noticed it wasn't getting better. I asked my mom, "Is Deb alright?" with a strange look on my face.

"She went to the emergency room today, and they told her that she got bronchitis," she said. "They gave her some medicine, so she'll be fine."

"Ok," I said as I walked away to my room hoping that what momma said was right and that she'll be back on her feet and smiling again. By April, she went to the doctor for the second time. She got her results, but before she could tell me, God told me first.

One morning I was tossing and turning. While in my dream, God kept showing me people I gained but got exchanged for another person in a golden ring of light. It was like he was playing out slides of all those I've loved and lost, but at the final slide he showed me my aunt with my father standing next to her.

On the inside of the dream, my heart wept, but I didn't know on the outside of the space my body cried full tears as well, and I woke up saying "No!"

I pushed myself out of bed. I slowly opened the door from my room to head to the kitchen and found my aunt with her head in her hands above her Bible and my mother rubbing her back for comfort.

Face still wet from the tears, I said, "Is there something you need to tell me?" Within a breath, my mom said, "Deb has Stage 4 lung cancer." My heart sank further because for this one time I wanted my dreams to be wrong.

I walked up to her with a smile and said, "We're going to beat this, and you're going to be just fine, but until then, what do you want your victory dinner to be?" I smiled, and it brought a chuckle to her face. "We can do some collard greens, deviled eggs, some mac 'n cheese, whatever you want!" I said in my funny southern accent. She laughed, I hugged her and told her, "I love you momma." Her reply: "I love you too Ariel."

Not long after getting news of Deb's diagnosis, her son Jeremy and daughter Deandrea were the first ones to stop by the house. Soon after came my Aunt Ann with her children Zarra and Marcus. It felt like a mini family reunion, plus it was the most people I've seen in the house in years. It was good to see us all together, but I wish it were under better circumstances. As we geared up for the fight for her, Ann led us in prayer, and to start our journey for this challenge, she poured anointed oil on all our hands. We started to pray as a family.

A lot of things shifted from that point in the house. The doctor ordered an electric bed for Deb because her current bed was too high for her to get down from since she'd be starting radiation treatments. Thankfully, chemo was ruled out in her situation.

We all took turns taking her to treatment. In addition, mom, Jeremy, Dee and I took turns helping her with her breathing treatments and medication. I even made a schedule as to when she took her medication and breathing treatments for the nurse.

My mother would bathe Deb while Jeremy or I would put her on the pot if she needed to use the restroom. When she couldn't eat much due to the radiation, we'd supplement her meals with boost shakes but always kept water by her side.

During this time, I believe we were on the right path to recovery for her, but certain aspects of my life took a hit consequently.

I fell behind on homework as my focus was dedicated to ensuring she received all the support she needed. This forced me to make a decision that would not only affect my personal ambitions but also signified my commitment to her well-being.

When next semester rolled around, I contacted my academic advisor to disclose to him that I wouldn't be coming back that term due to family obligations. Though uncertain of my return, I told him that I would keep him updated when I could resume my studies where I left off.

Simultaneously, my relationship with my boyfriend Terry of two years faced strains due to my increased responsibilities at home. Fortunately, he understood because he knew how important family was to me and stood by me. Our planned trip to Myrtle Beach for my birthday in September remained uncertain until we knew the progress of Deb's health. Until then we agreed to stay connected through video chat every two weeks.

The first night proved challenging for her as the current bed arrangement left her unable to sleep comfortably. Opting for the recliner in the living room, I vividly recall the sound of the leather as she adjusted amidst the pillows that surrounded her. I grabbed my blanket and pillow, settling on the small couch nearby, prepared just in case she needed me. "You need to get some rest for work tomorrow; you go on to bed, I'll be fine," Deb insisted. "I'm OK. I'm not sleeping until you get some sleep," I reassured her.

Despite her protests, she didn't argue further and adjusted enough to eventually nod off. This wasn't the first night I'd have to stay up with her. On a previous occasion, she had called me from my room after I had just returned from the bathroom. I could see her restlessness and asked her if she needed anything. She asked me to pray for her.

As I stood by her side, I asked God to grant her peace, dispel her fears for a tranquil sleep and give her strength to walk independently each day. Once I knew she was sound asleep, I whispered, "I love you," before retiring to bed.

As the summer began, I was excited for our family trip to Blacksville, S.C., to God's Acre Healing Springs. This well was known for its healing properties, and our tradition involved bringing along our empty water bottles, milk bottles or jugs in bags to fill up with water for the season. Our hope was that this direct connection with God's healing waters would contribute to Deb's recovery.

This water had aided many others, and it was always so refreshing to drink. On a scorching July morning, our journey commenced at 10 a.m. with the goal of arriving before the crowds. By 11 a.m., we reached the springs, ready to fill our containers.

I jumped out of the car to assist Deb, positioning myself by her side in case she needed support, but with the aid of her cane and assistance from Jeremy, she got out safely. As we approached the spring, Deb, stood before the double spout leaning on it without her cane crying out to God. My aunt Ann stood behind her, rubbing her back to comfort her while praying on her behalf. This moment by far was the hardest for me because I personally wished I could snap my fingers to make her better, but I knew I wasn't God and it wasn't something I had the power to control, but it never hurts to dream.

As the weeks went by, summer came and went before we knew it. We were back into the cooler months again. During this time, though the pandemic ravaged the world, during all that there were some uplifting moments: my birthday was a couple days away with a chance that I could take a break from being the medical personnel on duty.

Dee brought Deb her lo mein noodles from her favorite Chinese restaurant, and earlier that day she used her walker to independently make it to the bathroom by herself. That's the first time since she'd been bed bound that she did something on her own. I cried when I saw her progress because that was my sign of hope that there would be nothing to worry about while I was gone.

On the day of my departure for Myrtle Beach, I double checked on mama to make sure she'd be fine without me there. My cousin Jeremy stayed over that weekend as precaution, and if they needed me, I was only a phone call away.

When October rolled around, we noticed Deb wouldn't eat anything but rather drank boost shakes and water and ate ice. Not long after that she didn't want to get out of bed besides using the pot and go back to bed.

She'd become so weak that the muscles in her leg became atrophied. We told Nurse Debra, and after a visit from the doctor, they told us there was nothing else we could do but enjoy our last days with her, however many there were.

With each passing day I tried to pray and ask God, "Did I do enough? Did I not pray enough? So why was this happening?!"

I stepped back for a second because I didn't want my frustration to show. I took a deep breath, and I stepped outside to check myself. I called Terry to let him know what the nurse told us. Without hesitation he came over to be by my side.

On Oct. 16, 2020, I was called in to do a delivery for the nursing home I was contracted to work. Deb was breathing from the oxygen machine, and my mom was tidying up in her room.

I had packed my lunch in my bookbag for the road, but before I left, I went to visit her. She seemed so cold, but I wanted her to know that I was here. I leaned over and whispered saying, "I love you mama; I'll see you when I get off" as I kissed her forehead and went to work.

Terry kept me company on my delivery stops. He knew my mind was still on Deb, but he still tried to cheer me up anyway. I finished my last delivery in Aiken, S.C., at about 11 p.m. and stopped by the gas station to fill up before heading home.

Before we could pull off, my phone rang. My heart started to drop when I saw it was my mother, and for a split second all I wanted to do was hide because I was afraid of what was coming next.

Without hesitation, I picked up the phone shaking, "Hey Mom," but before I could finish the sentence that's when she said Deb was gone. She died at about 10:30 p.m., not long after I left for work.

It took me a moment to process what she said, and the only thing I felt was all the emotions from the journey. I got out of the car and kicked the tire multiple times, cried and screamed as loud as I could.

It felt like someone had ripped my heart out of my chest. It was the same feeling I had when my father had passed, and just like that day my life wouldn't be the same.

I write this story to tell you that although she passed on, we wanted to send the message as a family that love never returns void, her love for us gave us the strength and resilience to give that love back ten-fold, and I hope you can do the same with those you love.

# 14

# EMBRACING THE PAIN & DIFFICULTY OF CANCER

## BY TERRY TUCKER

Many people mark their lives based on the highs and lows they experience. For example, they view weddings, graduations and promotions as the good times, and funerals, layoffs and health issues as the bad times. We use these measuring events because extremes tend to remain with us.

But it's the day-in and day-out courageous fight that we put up when we are tired, scared or hurting where the real battle of life is won.

My life has been no different, especially when it comes to my experience with cancer. While I had three of my four grandparents die of malignancies, they passed late in life, most likely due to contributing lifestyle factors such as smoking, poor diet or being sedentary.

However, the first time cancer impacted me directly was shortly after I graduated from college. Being the first person in my family to graduate from college, I was all set to make my mark on the world with my newly obtained business administration degree. Since this was a time long before the internet was available to help people find jobs, I moved home to look for employment. After months of sending out numerous resumes and going on countless dead-end interviews, I was fortunate to land a position in the marketing department at the corporate headquarters of Wendy's International, the fast-food restaurant chain, just outside Columbus, Ohio. That was the good news.

The bad news was that, unfortunately, a few months after starting at Wendy's, my 82-year-old grandmother, who was living with us, developed lymphoma, and several months later we learned that my 51-year-old father had end-stage breast cancer.

While having two family members in the same household inflicted with a terminal disease was certainly tragic, it especially impacted my mother. Literally in bedrooms side-by-side to one another, her mother and her husband were slowly giving up the ghost.

Over the next 3.5 years, our family unified to provide continuous care and support to these family members who we knew were not going to recover. A few years after my grandmother was diagnosed, she succumbed to her cancer, and 18 months later, we were back at the same cold, gloomy and windy cemetery laying my father to rest.

Living at home and sleeping in the same twin bed I had grown up in was not how I planned to spend the years immediately after college. But it did afford me the opportunity to have many deep, meaningful and poignant conversations with my father. Those talks provided a depth of soul regarding the meaning of life, the importance of family and the moral obligation we all have to find our purpose in life while we are healthy, strong and energetic.

Watching my big, heroic and resilient father waste away as cancer consumed his body was certainly difficult and painful, but it taught me the lesson of ensuring you have a purpose when dealing with adverse and difficult times in your life.

Standing by the open grave witnessing my father's body being returned to the earth, I recalled how much he impressed upon me the need to have a mission in hard times. As I turned from the family plot and was buffeted by the balmy winds whipping among the headstones, I tucked that important message in the back of my mind for the day when I would face my mortality.

Ironically, like my father, the greatest challenge of my life began in early 2012 when I was 51 years old. I was a girl's high school basketball coach in Texas when I had a callus break open on the bottom of my left foot. Since being a coach requires you to be on your feet for many hours a day for practices and games, I initially didn't give the wound much thought.

After a few weeks of the callus not healing, I went to see a podiatrist friend of mine who took an X-ray and determined I had a cyst within the wound. He explained he could cut it out, which he did. After the minor surgery, he showed me the transparent gelatin sac with a white fatty substance inside. He assured me that everything looked normal but that he would send the growth off to pathology to confirm his benign diagnosis.

Two weeks later, I received a call from my friend letting me know that the innocuous nodule inside my callus, which raised no concern when it was removed, was a rare and deadly form of cancer called Acral Lentiginous Melanoma. He further raised my anxiety level by telling me that in the 25 years he had been practicing medicine, he had *never* seen this form of cancer. Because my cancer was so rare, he recommended I be treated at the world-renowned M.D. Anderson Cancer Center in Houston, Texas.

At M.D. Anderson, I had two surgeries to remove the tumor and the lymph nodes in my groin and had a skin graft to close the wound on the bottom of my foot where the melanoma was excised.

At the time of my diagnosis, I was told that melanoma was a death sentence, and the only treatment option the doctors could offer me was surgery. If the cancer emerged in an area where they could cut it out, they would. Otherwise, there was no other therapy they could provide me.

If I received a miracle, I was told I might live five years, but more than likely, I'd be dead within two years. I took the doctor's prognosis with a measured response. While they knew the odds of how long a person with my type of cancer might live, they didn't know my heart, they didn't understand my mind, and they didn't comprehend the power of my soul. I had a wonderful family, a great job and a purpose larger than anyone understood. There was plenty to live for.

I decided to take the death sentence I was given and turn it into a life sentence. How much living could I squeeze into whatever amount of time I had left, while still working with my medical team to combat the cancer?

When I healed from the surgeries, I was put on a weekly injection of the drug Interferon to keep the disease from returning. My oncologist described this medication as, "kicking the can down the road," buying me as much time as possible for additional therapies to become available to treat melanoma.

Interferon therapy was a horrible, nasty and debilitating experience. I lost 50 pounds during my treatment. I was constantly nauseous, fatigued and chilled. My ability to taste food had significantly diminished, and my body continually ached. This misery went on for over 1,660 days until the Interferon became so toxic to my body that I ended up in the intensive care unit with a body temperature of 108 degrees, which usually isn't compatible with being alive. Somehow, I survived the Interferon toxicity but had to stop taking the medicine.

One thing I learned during all my pain and discomfort is that you have two choices: you can succumb to the debilitating discomfort and misery, or you can learn to embrace it and use it to make you a stronger and more resilient human being. I chose the latter.

Please understand that there were days I felt so poorly and was in so much agony that I prayed to die. I just wanted out of this life. I didn't feel I was living; I was just not dying. Each day was a struggle to use my mind to override the apathy and distress my body was feeling.

I was no better at dealing with pain and discomfort than the next person. But every day, I found a way to survive, with the knowledge I would need to do it again the following morning.

Almost immediately after stopping the Interferon, the melanoma returned in the exact same spot on my foot where it had presented five years earlier in 2012.

This necessitated the amputation of my left foot in 2018. While losing my foot was certainly tragic, I considered myself lucky. The reason I felt fortunate was that the initial discussion with my oncologist and orthopedic surgeon recommended a below-the-knee amputation.

Fortunately, with a collaboration between my orthopedic surgeon and a foot specialist, they were able to perform a Lisfranc amputation, which removed everything in front of my ankle, which were the metatarsals and transmetatarsals.

While I needed an insert in my shoe and physical therapy to learn to walk again, this process was much easier and faster since I still had the use of my ankle and heel.

In the summer of 2019, I felt a small nodule in the middle of my left shin. When I showed it to my oncologist, he didn't think it was cancer, but given my history, ordered the lump biopsied. Sure enough, it turned out the be another melanoma tumor.

Once again, I found myself back under the surgeon's scalpel having a portion of my shin removed. With the surgical margins clean, meaning the outer edge of the tissue that was taken was free of cancer, I thought I might have some time to rest and recover.

Since up to this point the cancer had been isolated to my left leg, shortly before the holidays in 2019, the head of surgical oncology recommended I undergo a little-used treatment that was developed in the 1950s called isolated limb perfusion with the hope of killing the remaining cancer cells in my leg.

In conjunction with a vascular surgeon and while I was under general anesthetic, the blood supply to my leg was reduced using a tourniquet. An incision was made in my groin to expose the femoral artery and vein. Once the vessels were uncovered, a catheter was inserted in each one, and chemotherapy was circulated through my leg for approximately an hour. When the procedure was concluded the catheters were removed, the vessels were stitched, and the blood supply to my leg was re-established.

One of the down sides of the procedure was that I had to remain in the hospital for five days while I was monitored every two hours to ensure I had adequate blood profusion throughout the leg.

By early 2020, just as the COVID pandemic was getting underway, I developed, what my doctors thought was a hematoma in my ankle as a result of the isolated limb perfusion procedure. It was suspected the hematoma was causing lymphedema, or fluid to build up in my lower leg, and I was referred to an occupational therapist for treatment.

After several weeks of therapy from my amazing therapist, my fluid retention was getting worse and not better. My therapist was the first to raise the alarm by contacting my surgeon and suggesting something more was going on within my leg and recommending I be scanned.

My physician agreed and scheduled me for an ultra-sound. Unfortunately, the technician who performed the test was unable to get a conclusive reading from the procedure and recommended I receive a CAT scan.

During this time, I woke up one morning unable to walk on my left leg without tremendous pain in my lower shin. This new symptom relegated me to having to use a cane to get around.

On a brisk early morning in April 2020, I found myself lying on the hard CAT scan table at the UCHealth Highlands Ranch Hospital hoping this test would help my doctors identify the simple cause of why I was in so much pain when I walked and why the fluid in my leg was not responding to treatment.

Around three o'clock that afternoon, I received a call from my oncologist with the sobering news. The reason I was having so much trouble walking was because what we thought was a hematoma in my ankle was actually a sizeable melanoma tumor that had grown large enough to fracture my tibia.

As if that wasn't bad enough, my doctor informed me that my entire lower leg was filled with cancer and would need to be amputated above the knee. The icing on the cake was his assertion that I also had large tumors in both lungs and fluid buildup around the pleural spaces of each lung.

To say I was devastated by this news would have been an understatement. I had gone into the CAT scan that morning thinking there was an easy explanation for my inability to walk comfortably, and a few hours later I was told my leg would need to be amputated above the knee and I had large tumors in both lungs. In addition, COVID had shut down all elective medical procedures, which caused a slight delay in having the amputation because my surgeon had to get special permission to perform the operation.

Five days after receiving this crushing news, my wife dropped me off at the hospital for my amputation. Again, because of COVID, I was not allowed to have anyone with me for the operation. My wife asked me what she should do during the surgery, and I suggested she just wait in the parking lot and pray until she received a call from my orthopedic surgeon.

After getting out of the car and into a wheelchair, a nurse pushed me into the pre-op area that was split into 30 bays, all designed to prepare patients for different surgeries. I was the only patient in this cavernous room, and the silence was deafening.

As I was prepped for surgery by the nurse and an anesthesia resident, my fear and anxiety continued to mount. At one point, I just wanted to run from the room, but with a broken leg, I knew this was impossible.

After a quick visit from my surgeon and anesthesiologist to go over the paperwork and sign the consent forms, I was given an injection of the drug Versed, which helped calm my anxiety.

When I was wheeled into the operating room, I had the anesthesiologist and one of the nurses help me sit up. I wanted to glance around the room and take one final look at the leg that had betrayed me for the past eight years and would shortly no longer be part of me.

I was supposed to stay in the hospital for 10 to 14 days after the operation to learn how to function with only one leg. However, due to the threat of the COVID infection, I was sent home with a freshly amputated limb after 48 hours. Fortunately, my occupational thera-pist agreed to visit our home after work on the day I was discharged from the hospital to help my wife set up the house for a person using a walker and wheelchair. The doorways in our home are too narrow for a wheelchair so I have to transition to a walker any time I want to go into a bedroom or bathroom.

Once I was rehabilitated from my amputation, my oncologist wanted to put me on chemotherapy to combat the tumors in my lungs. When I asked him if it would save my life, he replied, "Prob-ably not, but it might buy you some more time."

While I was healing after my surgery, I went with my wife to the mortuary, cemetery and church and planned my funeral. I was eight years into this cancer journey and not afraid to die because I believed I had lived the purposes I was put on this earth to do.

I explained to my doctor that I didn't want to take chemotherapy given that I was going to die anyway. However, I told him I would talk it over with my family and get back to him.

I was quite surprised when my wife and daughter were adamant that I take the chemotherapy. Although I didn't want to, I remem-bered something I learned when I was in the police academy in 1997: "You will fight harder for the people you love than you will fight for yourself." So, I took the chemotherapy not because I wanted to but because I loved my family more than I loved myself.

In hindsight, the chemotherapy treatments were the right course of action because they were the bridge that got me to the clinical trial drug I am on today that has kept the tumors in my lungs stable for the past three years.

One of my infusion nurses recently asked me what it was like to have my foot amputated in 2018 and my leg removed in 2020. I told her it hasn't been easy. Learning to walk again when you're 60 years old has not been easy. I further explained that cancer can take all my physical facilities, but it can't touch my heart, it can't touch my mind, and it can't touch my soul. And that's who we really are.

We know this body will die and decay, but our hearts, minds and souls are eternal and will live on. If cancer has taught me anything, it's that in the daily battle against the disease, the most important thing I can focus on is using my malignancy to harden my mind, open my heart and strengthen my soul.

With those three things nourishing my life, regardless of the outcome, I win in the end.

# WHAT'S NEXT?

Want to stay up to date on the latest Showing Up: Perspectives On Cancer shows, events, books and more? Go to Perspectiveson Cancer.com to sign up for our email newsletter.

**Subscribe to our YouTube Channel** to watch shows with many of the authors in this book - and more.

Want to be a guest or a sponsor on Showing Up: Perspectives On Cancer? Email tim@sohnsocialmediasolutions.com to be considered.

Made in United States
North Haven, CT
12 April 2024